Kodansha America, Inc.
114 Fifth Avenue, New York, New York 10011, U.S.A.

Kodansha International Ltd.
17-14 Otowa 1-chome, Bunkyo-ku, Tokyo 112, Japan

Published in 1995 by Kodansha America, Inc.

Copyright © 1995 by Mitchell L. Gaynor, M.D.
All rights reserved.

The author gratefully acknowledges the following sources of quotations:

From Tales of the Hasidim *by Martin Buber. Copyright © 1947 and copyright renewed © 1975 by Schocken Books, Inc., a division of Random House, Inc.*

From Ten Rungs: Hasidic Sayings, *by Martin Buber. Copyright © 1947 by Schocken Books, Inc., a division of Random House, Inc.*

Number Seven from "The Way of Life According to Laotzu" from The Chinese Translations *by Witter Bynner. Copyright © 1944 by Witter Bynner and copyright renewed © 1972 by Dorothy Chauvenent and Paul Horgan. Reprinted by permission of Farrar, Straus & Giroux, Inc.*

Thomas Merton: The Way of Chuang Tzu. *Copyright © 1965 by The Abbey of Gethsemani, Inc. Reprinted by permission of New Directions Publishing Corp.*

Library of Congress Cataloging-in-Publication Data

Gaynor, Mitchell L., 1956–
Healing essence : a cancer doctor's practical program for hope
and recovery / Mitchell L. Gaynor.
p.   cm.
Includes bibliographical references.
ISBN 1-56836-079-7
1. Cancer—Alternative treatment.   2. Mind and body therapies.
3. Visualization.   4. Cancer—Psychosomatic aspects.   I. Title.
RC262.G38   1995
616.99'406—dc20   95-18162

Book design by Margaret M. Wagner

Printed in the United States of America

95 96 97 98 99 Q/FF   10 9 8 7 6 5 4 3 2 1

To my mother
who showed me how strength and surrender
could so beautifully coexist

To my wife
whose light and inner compass have faithfully
provided me with invaluable direction and
guidance

To my son
who by the time he was two gave me a far
greater perspective on life than I
had ever known

To my father
for always being there

This is my secret, it is very simple. You can only see well with your heart. The essence of things is invisible to the eyes.
—*Antoine de Saint-Exupéry,*
The Little Prince

What you should put first in all the practice of our art is how to make the patient well; and if he can be made well in many ways, one should choose the least troublesome.
—*Hippocrates*

Contents

Part Three: THE FOUR PATHS OF HEALING MEDITATION

The patients involved have given me consent to use the clinical vignettes in this book. To protect their privacy, I have changed names, transposed events, merged the stories of different people, and altered identifying characteristics.

The guided imagery techniques in this book are not substitutes for professional medical care. Because everyone is different, a physician must diagnose individual conditions and supervise all health problems. I urge you to seek out the best medical resources available to help you make informed decisions.

"E.S.S.E.N.C.E." is the abbreviation and acronym for Dr. Gaynor's unique seven-step "experience, see, surrender, empower, nurture, create, and embody" program described in this book. Both "E.S.S.E.N.C.E. GUIDED IMAGERY" and "EGI" are proprietary marks of Dr. Gaynor for meditative healing. For enhanced readability, the seven periods have been omitted from "E.S.S.E.N.C.E." as it appears in the text.

Healing
ESSENCE

Introduction

As a cancer doctor, I see suffering every day. But I also see miracles of healing. These are miracles performed by people who use their own inner power to transform themselves spiritually and physically. This book is about the inner power these people awake in themselves.

As I became increasingly aware of the healing power deep within myself and within others, I tried to find some message or signal to make my patients aware of it, too. However, I found this was easier said than done. What actually happened was that my patients became my teachers. Those who had recovered against the odds and against medical prognostications already had what I was seeking. So I went to them.

People who had *proved* their remarkable healing power by participating in their own recovery all had one thing in common: they had an awareness of their *soul, essence,* or *inner being* (I use those terms interchangeably)—although that doesn't mean they were necessarily religious. And I learned from them that awareness of our essence—awareness alone—is enough to set the healing process in motion.

Hippocrates, the Greek physician often called the father of medicine, said that nature heals and that the physician is only nature's attendant. So to help people, including myself, recognize and use this healing essence, I put together a program called ESSENCE Guided Imagery. My approach involves state of the art medical science, nutritional evaluation, counseling, dream awareness, and guided imagery. This book concentrates on guided imagery techniques and meditations you can do on your own.

A patient in my practice receives treatment in four basic ways. First, a physician defines and thoroughly investigates the person's immediate physical problem. The physician then outlines a treatment plan, using the best therapies known. Second, nutritional strategies are employed. (At the Strang-Cornell Gastrointestinal Cancer Prevention Center, I study the link between nutrition, diet, and vitamins in cancer prevention and treatment.) Third, counseling of the person is essential. Past traumas that may have contributed to the illness are discussed; fears, guilt, and dreams are explored. Fourth, the person uses guided imagery, meditations, and paths such as those outlined in this book to focus his or her own healing power.

Thus, my integrated, comprehensive approach ignores none of the many aspects of the healing process. In this sense, it is holistic. Many practitioners of holistic medicine, however, have embraced "alternative medicine" *exclusively.* This is where my approach differs. I fully believe in the power of modern medicine—although I also believe that it is not the be-all and end-all. My experience is that when all aspects of the healing process can be integrated, a radical shift occurs in the way patients view medical professionals and in the way doctors view their practices.

Healing occurs on several levels. The body heals on a physical level, and this can involve the use of traditional medical treatments such as antibiotics, surgery, and chemotherapy, as well as other nontraditional methods such as acupuncture, massage, and diet. But treating a patient on the physical plane alone is like fixing a leaky roof by drilling a hole in the floor. Healing must also address *why* an illness or depression developed. On this level, healing is not so much concerned with "fixing" the symptom as with asking what truth is being ignored or what unconscious aspects of the patient are being neglected. Frequently, the symptoms reflect messages the person's inner being is trying to convey. Illness is sometimes the only way this essence can balance its emotional energy and can jar a person into noticing something.

Patients with cancer feel a range of emotions upon learning of their diagnosis. Fear, anger, and sadness are among the most common. Such reactions are understandable and lead to what I call a sense of *disconnectedness* from both the higher self and the world. A world that allows the misfortune of cancer, many patients conclude, is one that they neither feel connected to nor desire to be a part of. Reestablishing this connection is critical for the healing process to thrive. A comprehensive approach to patient care is necessary to establish links between patients, their world, and their higher self. Nutritional support that enhances one's sense of physical well-being automatically reestablishes a feeling of connectedness to the earth from which this nutrition comes.

I developed guided meditations as part of the ESSENCE process to help my patients become aware of their fears about illness and to bring healing into their lives. The name *ESSENCE* comes from the first letter of each of the seven steps involved in the process. The steps, which are explained more fully in Part Two, are as follows:

1. Experience
2. See
3. Surrender
4. Empower
5. Nurture
6. Create
7. Embody

These seven steps allow you to experience your higher self by asking your own questions.

You do not have to be sick to benefit from the ESSENCE Guided Imagery process. By practicing this process, you become aware of your inner being. The process can also help you heal the fear, depression, sadness, and suffering all of us have experienced.

Through ESSENCE healing you can begin to overcome these negative emotions by discovering what life means and how to live life aligned with your higher self.

In Part One, I describe how, as a young doctor, I came to realize that there was much more to healing than the information in medical textbooks suggested. What the textbooks never told me was that people have the power to assist in their own healing. When we look at how people become aware of their hidden inner healing power, we see that these are ordinary people, like you and me, who do not have lofty thoughts or visions. Yet they—and you and I—possess inner powers that conventional medicine is only now beginning to acknowledge.

In Part Two, I introduce the ESSENCE process and guide you through the seven steps toward healing physical discomfort. Also, I describe a guided meditation to remove the barriers to healing.

In Part Three, I describe the four kinds of guided meditation, or paths, that are part of the ESSENCE process. The four paths are (1) healing fear, (2) going beyond suffering, (3) ending melancholy, and (4) creating hope.

In Part Four, I guide you through a 28-Day Healing Journey, which is a day-by-day guide that follows each of the four paths in turn over a period of four weeks. This journey in the mind can help bring you spiritual and physical rejuvenation. I also discuss a variety of other ways to connect with your inner life.

Our bodies are designed to experience health. Even down to the cellular level, our bodies are continually working to maintain homeostasis, or a striving for balance and well-being. ESSENCE Guided Imagery is designed to make you aware of the power of your inner being so that you can always experience healing. It is also a path of finding healing by accepting whatever adversity you may be experiencing, so that this adversity forms a base from which you not only can grow but also can discover and recover your inner power.

Healing is a path that must be traveled, a journey to be experienced. In this book I do not try to *tell* you what inner healing is. Instead, I give techniques for *discovering* the healer within yourself. The instant you discover what inner healing is, you begin to be healed.

The purpose of this book, then, is to help you expand your awareness of the possibilities of the healing process. The ESSENCE steps allow you to remove the barriers to healing. But the power of this healing is not in the process. The power lies within you.

Part One

Essence
and Healing

1

Understanding Our Essence

One summer day when I was twelve, I saw Fernando Dominguez at a tree near our house. He was talking to it and shaking it gently with both hands.

Dominguez, as he liked to be called, was a Pueblo Indian who had left his homeplace years earlier because of impoverished conditions and lack of work. He did yard work for my father at our house and at my father's dental office in Plainview, Texas, a farming community just below the Panhandle. They say you can see farther and see less in Plainview than anywhere else.

"Your father asked me to cut this tree down, but it's not dead yet," Dominguez said. He told me that he could see the essence in any living thing, and so long as it still had essence, it wasn't dead. Although the tree looked dead to me, Dominguez continued to water it, talk to it, and shake it daily. Over the next month, it developed buds and, later, leaves. Today, many years later, the tree is alive and healthy. It was from Dominguez that I first heard the word *essence* used in this way.

One day, Dominguez did not show up for work. After not having heard from him for an entire week, my father called the police and found he had been picked up in a farmer's field "talking to himself and acting crazy." He had been committed to the state psychiatric hospital in Big Spring. My father never turned down an opportunity to help another person, especially those who could not help themselves, so he took a day off work and drove to the psychiatric institution. The administrator listened to my father explain that Dominguez, in spite of talking to plants, worked regularly and never hurt anyone. He was released into my father's custody several days later.

Dominguez told me about his week in the psychiatric hospital. "Your society is even more barbaric to your own people than it has been to mine," he said. "You have taken our land, but you have not taken our spirit. But your own people who see beyond the visible—you lock them up and break their spirit."

His eyes, dark and seeking, looked into mine. "How will you keep them from breaking your spirit?" he asked.

"I don't understand," I stammered.

"You will need protection," he told me.

I may have guessed that this proud man, who was poor monetarily, was seeking to repay my father through a gift to his son. Certainly, I was already aware Dominguez knew things that no one else in town did, including my father.

After thinking for a while, Dominguez said, "Tell me more about that place you go camping with your friends."

I had gone on several Boy Scout camping trips to Palo Duro Canyon, about fifty miles away. Afterward, I had shown Dominguez arrowheads I had found, and no doubt had described my stirring adventures there. He knew that this wild place was special to me and that I was always ready to talk about exploring it further.

"How about you and I go on a weekend campout there?" he asked when I finished the tale of my latest adventure.

My father consented, but only for a weekend. After my father had dropped us at the main camping area, said good-bye, and driven off, Dominguez said, "Let's start walking. We have a long way to go."

I asked why we couldn't leave our camping gear where we were.

"I can't show you anything here," he said. "There are too many people."

We hiked into the hills and set up camp on a ledge on a canyon wall outside the entrance to a small cave. When I looked down, I could see the whole canyon spread out beneath me.

"I thought I knew every inch of this place," I said. "I never knew you could get up here. Have you been here a lot?"

"I've never been here before," Dominguez replied.

We made a fire. As darkness fell, the stars filled the sky.

Dominguez said, "Tonight you'll stay here alone. I'll be back in the morning. Is that okay?"

Not wanting to seem afraid, I told him it was fine.

"I want you to do something—don't ask the reason," he said. "I want you to look up at the stars tonight and loudly insult them and criticize them. Then I want you to listen. Listen with your ears as well as your eyes."

Hoping my actions would help keep cougars, bears, and rattlers away, I bellowed every nasty word I knew at the stars. They just kept on twinkling up in the sky. I must have fallen asleep, for I awoke with the sun rising and feeling a hand on my shoulder. It was Dominguez.

"Did you do it?" he asked.

"Yes," I said.

"And what did the stars say to you?" he asked with a smile.

"Nothing," I admitted, "but the more I yelled, the more calm the stars seemed to become."

We ate breakfast and hiked around the canyon all day. I showed him all the special things I knew there: where to find arrowheads and geodes, and where to see beautiful rock formations. As it was getting dark, we cooked dinner on a fire back at the ledge.

"Tonight," Dominguez told me, "you will be alone again. Only this time, I want you to praise and compliment the stars loudly and listen with both your ears and your eyes for their response."

I did my best and at some point fell asleep. When he woke me the next morning, Dominguez again asked if I had done what he had instructed. I said I had.

"And how did the stars reply?" he asked.

I shook my head regretfully. "Nothing. But I did feel them become even more peaceful," I added as an afterthought.

"Good," he replied. "You have begun your path with a most important lesson."

Puzzled I looked at him. I was not aware of having learned anything.

"Be like the stars—like all of nature," he explained. "When you are criticized, answer only with calmness. And when you are praised, answer only with peacefulness. You see, the moment another's criticism is more important than his praise is, that is the moment you have lost your power—because you have lost touch with your essence."

He asked me if I understood his words.

"Sort of," I answered.

"Don't tell anyone about this until you fully understand it," he said. "If you do, it will lose its meaning."

Poverty had forced Dominguez from his pueblo, but he did not forget the ancient, honored ways of his people. Many of us have lost cultural traditions that emphasize our inner life, and we have been separated from our roots so long that we cannot go back to what might remain. The twentieth century has cut such a wide swath of change around the globe that the old pathways to spiritual life often have been obliterated. We may now have to make our own way, frequently in surroundings that discourage this kind of effort. Many of us are not even sure what we seek, and that must be our first concern.

DEFINING ESSENCE

Living life without an awareness of it having a deeper, more meaningful purpose and truth may lead to a variety of maladies, from depression to physical illness. Certainly, not all disease can be directly attributed to this lack of awareness. Viruses, physical accidents, genetic disorders, and many other illnesses are beyond our control. It is well documented, however, that our immune systems can be depressed by our attitudes and moods. In fact, a recent study in the British medical journal *Lancet* described a significant depression in T-lymphocyte counts in people who had been laid off their jobs (these so-called T-cells are part of the immune system's surveillance and defense system). There was also a correlation between the length of time the people had been laid off and the degree of depression of their T-cells.

The more we distance ourselves from the essence at the core of our selves and beings, the more prone we are to illness, and the more difficult it is to discover our own power for healing. This separation makes it more difficult to recover from illness. An awareness of our soul must become as much a part of healing as drugs, surgery, and hospitals.

Most of us have limiting ideas that prevent us from realizing our own essence, our power for self-healing, and our abilities for self-renewal. We need to let go of our notions that healing can come only from outside ourselves. Medicines and surgery clearly have an important role in treating illness; however, true healing begins and is completed within each individual.

We can initiate and create healing in our lives only if we allow ourselves to feel and see that it is possible. We must recognize that our fear that healing is impossible for us, our belief that healing can be found only outside ourselves, and our assumption that our present reality is permanent and unchangeable are all nothing more than conditioned thought patterns, and that they are in fact thoughts conditioned by fear. We can then begin the healing process by becoming conscious of the miracles all around us. This kind of knowing and understanding is not attained through our eyes or minds. Rather, it is an understanding that comes through quiet meditation, when we allow ourselves to let go temporarily of who we think we are, and then listen to what our essence is trying to tell us.

On a camping trip, my family and I were awakened one night by a distant clap of thunder. My son, who was three, moved his sleeping bag close to mine and said, "Dad, I'm scared of the thunder." I told him he was afraid of it because he did not understand it, and I explained that it was just a noise coming from the clouds, which were far away. That seemed to satisfy him, but just then a much louder clap of thunder rang out. He jumped out of his sleeping bag into my arms and said, "Dad, I still don't understand thunder."

It is the same with understanding our essence, our deepest fears, and our innermost longings—we need an understanding that goes beyond the linear thinking of our rational minds and egos. When you use the ESSENCE meditations, the wall surrounding your power for healing will begin to crumble, as you discover the love and light that have always been within you.

ESSENCE AND OUR LIVES

How have you reacted to the "bad things" in life, such as tragedy, loss, criticism, sickness, or other adversity? What about the "good things," such as wealth, success, praise, and health? Do you carry the whole spectrum of negative emotional energy around with you? Or do you live your life with the positive energy that comes from a sense of fulfillment?

We must ask ourselves if we are doing what we most want to do, what we want to express and can do best. If we are unfulfilled, are empty inside, or suffer from a sense of failure, we must ask where and why, for much of the illness, depression, and pessimism in our society results from our failure to live up to the best within us. This stems from our inability to love ourselves and from a lack of awareness of our own talent, love, and passion.

The twentieth-century Russian philosopher G. I. Gurdjieff characterized the newborn child as pure *essence*. He meant, as did my friend Dominguez, that essence is our deepest and highest self, with all its inherent passions, longings, tastes, and potential. Some people refer to this as the "inner self," "soul," "human spirit," or "heart." Regardless of what you call it, your essence is who you really were when you entered this world and the person you must attempt to rediscover.

Many people begin losing touch with their essence when very young. As children, many of us had our joy and excitement invalidated by overzealous discipline and our tempers controlled through punishment. We were taught to behave calmly in the face of excitement and to keep quiet when we were upset or angry. With each of these lessons, we gradually lost touch with a bit more of our essence and became more separated from our soul. Many of us have wondered why we aren't happy at times we think we should be, and we are perplexed when our achievements do not bring us fulfillment. This happens because over time we have lost touch with our inner self.

Even so, our essence does not lie dormant for long. In fact, illness or depression is often a message from that inner self saying that the only way left for healing to occur is to become aware of the soul again. When we fail to respond to this message, we are, in effect, making ourselves sick.

Life force or life energy is the basis of traditional Eastern medicine. In Chinese, the word for it is *chi;* in Japanese, *ki.* This life energy is important for both the spirit and body. Traditional Chinese medicine teaches that this life energy enters the human body through the breath. Likewise, in Western culture, the spirit was originally regarded as an animating vapor infused through the breath. The word *spirit* is derived from the Latin *spirare* (to breathe) and *spiritus* (a breath). The Bible refers to this life force in Genesis: "Then the Lord God formed a man from the dirt of the ground and breathed into his nostrils a breath of life, thus the man became a living creature."

Chinese medicine teaches that when there is an imbalance of this life force or *chi,* illness results. The breathing exercises that I recommend at the beginning of each ESSENCE Guided Imagery meditation are designed to help the practitioner focus awareness on the breath.

ILLUSION AND PERSPECTIVE

Many people feel ashamed of their lives and daily routines, which seem meaningless or menial. If you wish to heal your life, however, you must understand that it is not your job or routine that causes a sense of shame or failure, but a negative set of assumptions about who you are and what you are supposed to be doing. Through counseling, meditation, and dream awareness, many of my patients have uncovered basic assumptions about who they are that developed when they were children. The resulting powerlessness and worthlessness many harbor deep inside their unconscious often give rise to the fear and guilt so pervasive in their lives.

The ESSENCE process is designed to help patients slowly shed light on such illusion, see how it is responsible for much of their feelings of negativity, and heal them. Illnesses and crises do not cause destructive and pessimistic thoughts and emotions; reactions to adversity do. With a change in perspective and realization of your true self, you can come to be happy and fulfilled, serving your fellow human beings through whatever you do. I have seen many of my patients discover, through the ESSENCE process, a deeper meaning and purpose in their lives, and in so doing, heal and transform themselves.

GLIMPSING ESSENCE

Many illnesses that affect the body and mind can be healed. But be prepared: not all healing is what we may expect it to be. We must approach the process with a mind open to the true meaning of healing, as well as its many ramifications and possibilities.

We experience a great deal in life with our hearts instead of our rational mind. Our mind, however, can be made receptive to the insight and perspective received through our heart. Once this occurs, we understand that our essence, right now, has the power to create for us the necessary perspective both to begin the healing process and to experience its own reality.

Our essence may express itself through the body in appearance and personality. From this perspective, many of the maladies of various organs described in medical literature for centuries may more accurately be described as expressions of the soul.

ESSENCE AND BELIEF

Carl Jung, the Swiss pioneer of psychiatry, said, "We can never finally know. I simply believe that some part of the human self or soul is not subject to the laws of space and time." I believe each of us has an eternal essence. This kind of knowledge cannot be conveyed by a book or a teacher, nor is it a reality that can be proved. It can, however, be experienced. It is an insight that must come from a willingness to understand through quiet meditation. This experience requires the ability to let go of much of your prior conditioning in order to know who you really are, why you are here, and what truth lies within your essence.

We are each born with an inner being, but without knowledge of it. When unaware of this essence, we merely exist—not *live*. When we simply exist, we attempt to find fulfillment through our ego and mind. By *ego,* I mean the person we think we are—the ambitious, the successful, the honest, the brilliant. Our ego is always searching and seeking. It may find success, money, or possessions, but it will never find the truth that lies within our essence. The ego's searchings can lead only to unhappiness, lack of fulfillment, and frustration, a pattern that makes us ignore even further our essence and the needs of our bodies.

Abraham Maslow, a pioneering psychologist in the human potential movement, has described the process of "self-actualization." This is the discovery of our potential for creativity, which lies within our essence. Those who live without going through this process struggle daily against their true self and the flow of life. We cannot carry on such a battle for long without draining ourselves of our energy, or becoming ill and depressed. But when we

achieve self-actualization and become aware of our essence, we realize that life is a continuing process of learning, loving, and
evolving.

But how can we discover the reality, as well as the richness, of
such an essence? To me, the following letter from Benjamin Franklin to a friend, Miss Hubbard, regarding the death of his brother,
John, truly demonstrates the insight and perspective of one who
has glimpsed his own essence and who understands healing in its
fullest sense.

Philadelphia, 22 February, 1756

I condole with you. We have lost a most dear and valuable
relation. But it is the will of God and nature that these mortal
bodies be laid aside when the soul is to enter into real life.
This is rather an embryo state, a preparation for living. A
man is not completely born until he be dead. Why, then,
should we grieve that a new child is born among the im-
mortals, a new member added to their happy society?

We are spirits. That bodies should be lent us while they
can afford us pleasure, assist us in acquiring knowledge, or in
doing good to our fellow-creatures, is a kind and benevolent
act of God. When they become unfit for these purposes and
afford us pain instead of pleasure, instead of an aid become
an encumbrance, and answer none of the intentions for which
they were given, it is equally kind and benevolent that a way
is provided by which we may get rid of them. Death is that
way. We ourselves, in some cases, prudently choose a partial
death. A mangled, painful limb which cannot be restored we
willingly cut off. He who plucks out a tooth parts with it
freely, since the pain goes with it; and he who quits the whole
body parts at once with all pains and possibilities of pains
and diseases which it was liable to or capable of making him
suffer.

Our friend and we were invited abroad on a party of pleasure which is to last forever. His chair was ready first and he is gone before us. We could not all conveniently start together, and why should you and I be grieved at this, since we are soon to follow and know where to find him?

Adieu,

B. Franklin

ESSENCE AND OPENNESS

True healing also needs to occur in the context of forgiveness, which allows us to accept the imperfections in our bodies and our lives. Before we can hope to have an experience of healing, we must be aware of our first reaction to illness. For most people, this is fear: fear of being unable to get what we want, fear of losing what we have, fear of losing control, fear of dying. ESSENCE imagery healing allows us to let go of our disappointment and anger when we are stripped of the pleasure and security to which we have become accustomed.

The truth that lies within our essence is revealed to us in glimpses. Some of these truths are simple: a child's laughter reminds us of our inherent innocence and natural joy; a walk in the park may remind us of our oneness with nature and its beauty; touching someone who is in pain brings out our natural compassion and helps us remember the joy in giving. Other truths are reflected in longings to create: to sing, write, teach, or heal. Many of these desires have previously been forced to lie dormant, suppressed for various reasons.

When the mind shuts out the truth within our essence, any endeavor—no matter how successfully executed and completed—becomes empty and meaningless. There are times we feel we have failed in life, no matter how much power, material wealth, sexual gratification, or religious experience we have acquired. We feel this way if our achievements lie outside the truth within our essence.

Carl Jung wrote, "Your vision will become clear only when you can look into your own heart." It is this clarity I have seen patients achieve when they embark on the ESSENCE journey, unleashing healing, joy, and love.

Bob: A Perspective on AIDS

▌Bob is a thirty-seven-year-old teacher who was referred to me two years ago with Kaposi's sarcoma, a type of skin cancer that occurs predominantly in patients infected with the HIV (AIDS) virus. He was married and had a two-year-old daughter. I informed him he needed to take an HIV test, given his diagnosis, and he agreed. My suspicions were confirmed—the test was positive. Both Bob and his wife were dumbfounded. "Here I am living my life, doing something I love, enjoying my family, and out of the clear blue this hits me," he said angrily. "How could this have happened to me?"

First, I gave Bob what he needed most—a shoulder to lean on and a kind ear to listen. Bob's helper lymphocyte count (a measure of his immune system) was very low, at a level of 34 (normal is over 400). This indicated a severe weakness in his immune system. He started taking the drug AZT to bolster his immune system, as well as chemotherapy for his cancer.

Bob's situation is not so different from the illnesses and patients I see daily. What is remarkable about Bob and his wife is their amazing transformation. On learning that he had tested HIV positive, Bob and his family were horrified. Bob and his wife began, somewhat reluctantly at first, to do the ESSENCE Guided Imagery meditations. After his first week of doing them twice daily, Bob told me that he was no longer afraid. "I've glimpsed who I am for the first time," he told me. "I didn't just have my heart broken; it was shattered. I wasn't affected by tragedy; I was overwhelmed with it. I felt totally immersed in sorrow at what I had been dealt. Then the thinking stopped. All of a sudden, I had perspective."

This perspective first emerged as a slew of questions. "Who defined for me what a long life is? What power do I have to contribute to my own healing? What does it feel like to know I'm powerless to change the past? If life is temporary, hadn't I better start asking what my purpose is and then live it?" Having perspective is different from "having all the answers." Perspective is attained by viewing life and its "problems" from one's essence. When viewed in this light, such conflicts and problems become far less negative. The result is a clarity that is far more calming and reassuring than so-called solutions or fixes.

Bob's wife also gained the perspective that ESSENCE healing brings. After two months of practicing, she told me, "I know that we are living in unique times. We can no longer assume that life is or will be a certain way. We all have to be grounded in who we are. I know that I can live just one day at a time and entrust the future to God."

Perspective is the first benefit of becoming aware of your essence.

Bob attained a complete remission from his cancer after six months of chemotherapy. His helper lymphocyte count has doubled. He lives his life one day at a time, never forgetting who he is. He still asks questions. He still learns. Bob still loves life, which is temporary for him—as it is for the rest of us.

2

Awakening the Healer in Ourselves

It is safe to say that every one of them fell ill because he had lost that which the living religions of every age have given to their followers.

—*Carl G. Jung,*
MODERN MAN IN SEARCH OF A SOUL

Healing is not found in medicines and surgery alone. While these are very important in treating illness, they are insufficient without the patient's participation in the process. Healing in its fullest sense requires looking into our heart and expanding our awareness of who we are.

Modern medicine tends to regard healing as coming only from outside us, overlooking the fact that we all have innate healing mechanisms, giving us the capability to be more than bystanders waiting for drugs and surgery to cure us. Adversity usually forces people to confront reality—and to do so without pretenses and other creations of the ego. Someone with serious illness usually has little concern for money, prestige, or position. And healing begins with the realization that with vulnerability comes a freedom from many of the illusions to which most of us are so attached. Many of my patients have used their own experiences with pain and vulnerability to make enormous leaps in their spiritual and psychological growth, and this relates closely to the entire healing process.

Ed: Strength to Deal with Hodgkin's Disease

▮ Ed was referred to me by his brother, a physician colleague of mine. Ed had Hodgkin's disease, a type of lymphatic cancer, that was advanced and involved nearly every lymph node in his body. He also had a serious blood infection and had lost thirty pounds. While hospitalized for two weeks, he received antibiotics and underwent aggressive chemotherapy to try to arrest the rapid spread of his cancer.

Able to express himself better through writing than speaking, he wrote me several letters, three of which I will share with you. They illustrate the healing and transformation described in this book. This is the first letter Ed sent me, shortly after he was discharged from the hospital:

7/8/89

Dear Dr. Gaynor:

Thank you for your kindness when I was in the hospital the last three weeks. The surgery and other treatments were hard and, I hope, over for a while. I am more scared now than anything else—not really for myself, but for my wife and two sons. My wife knows that I have advanced Hodgkin's disease and that I may have only a year or so. But what do I tell my ten-year-old? How do I tell him I may not be around to see him graduate from high school? How do I tell him I'm in too much pain to sit through his little league baseball games? And what about my six-year-old? He cried when I left for the hospital. I talked to him on the phone every day, and all he wanted to know was, "When are you coming home?" Now when I leave the house for tests, he cries and asks, "When are you coming home?" How do I tell him that one day daddy may never be coming home? It doesn't quite seem fair to any of us, but I guess life's like that sometimes.

I'll see you next week, Doc, and thanks for listening.

Sincerely, Ed

The following letter was written three months later, after I had instructed Ed in the ESSENCE Guided Imagery meditations:

10/12/89

Dear Dr. Gaynor:

I am writing this letter just after midnight. Joan and the children are asleep and I just completed a guided meditation. I can't thank you enough for teaching me the ways to touch my soul. I never knew so much power, such joy and such safety were always inside me. I started back to work last week, and to top it off, I now have a better job. I've gone from being ashamed for people to know I was sick to wanting to share the healing I've found with my friends at work. We all need healing; I was just fortunate enough to discover it. I now know one thing you may find hard to believe, but I realized just tonight. This came to me from a place deep inside. I am not going to die of cancer. I am going to beat it because I no longer need it in my life. I know you may not see it that way right now, but I'm sure you'll be open to it. I feel secure enough not to really worry about all the unimportant stuff either. When things come up, I know I can heal them too. I wish you and your family love and peace.

Ed

Three years after his initial diagnosis, I received the following letter from Ed:

7/26/92

Dear Dr. Gaynor,

I enjoyed seeing you again at my last appointment. You look better without a mustache. I knew I was still in remission but was pleased to hear your report confirming this anyway. I laugh whenever I think about your telling me of the radiologist asking, "What miracle drug did you give him?" when she saw my last gallium and CAT scan showing absolutely no disease. You answered, "I really didn't give him anything special." But the fact is you gave me everything. You gave me my life by showing me the way to healing. I have also been helping my family and friends come to know their own power to bring healing into their lives. I may never do this on your level, but it's my own small way of giving back what I have been given.

I want to share with you something I've never told anyone. Since I was about ten years old, I've said this prayer to God from time to time: "Please God, never let me get cancer." I figured I could handle most anything else—but after seeing my aunt and grandfather die of cancer, I figured I couldn't handle it. Now I know my prayer was answered. I learned I *can* handle it and I *did* handle it. It did it through trust, not doubt. It was doubt that caused me to fear it, and I know it was trust that allowed me to overcome it. I suppose saying thank you doesn't describe my gratitude, but I know you already know. See you in six months.

Ed

Ed's journey and that of many other patients I have had the privilege to care for began by taking a number of steps toward participating in his own healing. These are the steps that can also lead you to discover the power for healing within yourself. I am not advocating a type of "alternative medicine," nor am I proposing that the techniques and meditations in this book be used as an alternative to traditional medical practice. The tech-

niques and examples described are meant to be "additional medicine," not "alternative medicine." But I have found that the most
advanced chemotherapy is best tolerated and used by those patients
who are able to discover their own power for healing as well.

As of late 1994, Ed's recovery was holding strong.

HEALING AND THE SPIRIT

In medical school and residency, I learned about the physical reality we call our bodies. But it was from my patients that I learned
about the true nature and resilience of the human spirit. I also
learned how to help others arrive at a place within themselves that
is beyond fear and even beyond courage—a place of fearlessness.
It is there that the body, mind, and spirit connect with the healing
process.

I believe it is essential for medicine to return to its original
intention, which is the healing of body, mind, *and* spirit. However,
this intention must come from both doctors and patients, and it
requires that we open our mind and our heart to the power within
us—our essence.

HEALING AS AN ART

Many students go into medicine with the intent to become
physician-healers, yet they are never helped to understand what
true healing is. They enter medical school with an idealistic view
of the healing profession, wanting to learn not only about disease,
physiology, and anatomy, but also about the ancient *art* of healing.
But this latter desire receives little support in medical school, and
even less during internship and residency training, during which
patients are viewed as lists of problems to be solved in noncreative,
technical ways. When physicians carry this attitude into practice,
not only does the doctor–patient relationship suffer, but the doctor
and the patient suffer as individuals, too.

For example, during hospital rounds, I recently heard a patient described as "a thirty-four-year-old leukemic, with pneumonia and a low white blood count, whose current problems are a low potassium and new fever." None of the physicians there were aware that the same "thirty-four-year-old leukemic" was also worried about his wife and child, wanted to know why he had needed a blood transfusion the previous night, and would like to have known the names of the intern and resident who had examined him for five minutes earlier that morning.

While the objective care of a patient is an important part of medicine, it must not be allowed to overshadow the human part. A patient who needs *healing* is not like a car that needs fixing. Medicine has too often become only an objective description of symptoms and treatments. True healing has always been an art that focuses on the subjective in the patient's symptoms. A doctor who is concerned solely with objective symptoms and signs can talk only about lab results, chemicals, and numbers. These are important data *about* the patient, but alone, they do not completely *represent* the patient or provide the tools for healing. They do not convey the feelings, longings, and essence of the patient. To understand these, the doctor must be a healer. And only when intuition and feeling become as much a part of the physician as the rational mind does the physician become a healer. Healing requires that discovery and caring be part of the diagnosis and treatment of illness.

Similarly, relationships between doctor and patient too often stop short of compassion and richness. Doctors have become focused only on the problem-solving aspects of healing, on filling out insurance forms, complying with constantly changing Medicare guidelines, and providing information to "managed-care" coordinators. Unable to find spiritual satisfaction in their profession, physicians are also becoming disillusioned.

Hippocrates said, "Life is short, art long, the occasion fleeting, experience fallacious, and judgment difficult. The physician must not only be prepared to do what is right himself, but also to make the patient, the attendants, and the externals cooperate." Throughout history, many healers in the ancient tradition—Hippocrates, Maimonides, the sixteenth-century Swiss physician Paracelsus, and Carl Jung, among others—could heal both the body and the heart through a wisdom that is available only to people who have glimpsed the soul. Such an awareness is necessary for physical and psychological health.

Some of my colleagues are very dubious about such spiritual concepts. They cannot accept that there are aspects to healing that have nothing to do with physiology, drugs, or CAT scans. But medicine has forgotten its roots. With the increasing incidence of AIDS, tuberculosis that is resistant to medication, and cancer, healing with an awareness of the soul needs to be brought back into mainstream medicine and needs to be understood as part of traditional medicine.

MY OWN NEED FOR HEALING

My career has been one to which many other doctors have aspired. I have an academic appointment at one of the best teaching hospitals in the country and a Park Avenue practice. I was the chief of a chemotherapy unit at a major New York medical center, until I recently became the associate director of the Strang-Cornell Gastrointestinal Cancer Prevention Center. My training has been traditional and would be considered "the best." I graduated from a leading medical school and completed my internship and residency at one of the top U.S. medical centers. I became the chief resident in medicine, completed two fellowships, and have board certifications in one specialty and two subspecialties.

Yet despite training, position, and prestige, I have become more and more aware that something critical is missing in medicine today. I have also discovered I can give far more healing to patients than I had been taught I could as a medical doctor. And I have seen how miraculously patients have drawn on their own power for healing. But in having felt the loneliness, sadness, and pain that long hours of caring for patients with serious illness brings, I have also discovered my own need for healing.

PHYSICIAN, HEAL THY SON

When my son, Eric, was sixteen months old, he developed a progressive limp. I took him to one of the top orthopedic surgeons in New York, who, finding nothing wrong with his X-rays, suggested close observation. A week passed, and the limp worsened markedly. My wife and I, at the suggestion of our pediatrician, sought a second opinion from an orthopedic surgeon at a major teaching hospital. He found that our son's left ankle was swollen, but another series of X-rays showed nothing abnormal.

The following day, I was seeing a patient in my office when my secretary buzzed on the intercom and told me the pediatrician was on the phone.

"I got the results of Eric's blood tests today, and they are alarming," he said. "His white blood count is 22,000, almost all of which are lymphocytes, and his alkaline phosphatase is 4,000."

As a hematologist, I knew these results were far from normal and could have serious implications.

"I've arranged for Eric to see the chief of the Pediatric Leukemia Service at Sloan-Kettering," he said.

"How soon should Eric be seen?" I asked.

"Immediately."

I felt as if I had just stepped off a cliff. I asked myself, how could this happen to *my* son? As soon as my patient left, I cried in my office for about a minute. When I regained my composure, I phoned my wife at her workplace to ask her to meet me at Sloan-Kettering, had my secretary reschedule my appointments for the day, and went home to pick up Eric and his baby-sitter.

At Sloan-Kettering, the chief of the Pediatric Leukemia Service and I looked at a smear prepared from Eric's blood.

"With the other lab abnormalities and these atypical white blood cells, it may be leukemia," he said. "I'll have to do a bone marrow aspiration under general anesthesia in the morning to find out."

In an adult, this smear would definitely indicate leukemia. I tried to comfort my wife as best I could. Although he had just had four tubes of blood drawn after three needle sticks, Eric now seemed oblivious to the situation and was playing with a toy cow he had just been brought by one of my colleagues, whose office was across the street. But here was I, a doctor who dealt with the most serious illnesses and cared for the sickest patients, faced with the greatest shock and sadness of my life. I wondered sadly whether Eric would have to suffer through chemotherapy, injections, hair loss, bone marrow aspirations, and spinal taps—things I knew about far too well. My wife and I both prayed to God that night for strength and for Eric's health.

That evening I did an ESSENCE Guided Imagery meditation. A sense of surrender, the likes of which I'd never experienced, overcame me. "Yes," I told myself, "maybe my life will be caring for a sick child. Instead of taking him to movies and Disney World, maybe for the next four years we'll be going to emergency rooms and doctors' offices." With all the sadness of this realization, however, an amazing sense of acceptance and peace continued to remain with me.

We arrived at Sloan-Kettering promptly at 9:15 the following morning. I was struck by the variety of people in the waiting room, from men in overalls to women in expensive Chanel suits. The children were all adorable, even though their treatment meant many had bald heads and puffy faces. Eric's doctor ordered an IV and six more tubes of blood to be drawn. Eric cried more each time the technician missed the vein. It took three people, including myself, to hold him still. My wife and I held his hand as the anesthesiologist administered the medication to make him fall asleep. His little hands went limp and his head fell back. I felt like I was seeing my own child die in my arms.

The doctor came out twenty minutes later and told me that the procedure had gone well and that we should have a result in about two hours. As my wife and I were standing by Eric's stretcher after he woke up, a man in work clothes, whose three-year-old son was receiving chemotherapy, came over to me in the waiting area and said, "Don't worry about the pain from his IV. Tonight, they will put a Broviac catheter in him, so they don't have to keep putting in IV's for chemotherapy." I told him confidently that we hoped it would not be necessary, because the doctor had just done a bone marrow aspiration, and it might not even be leukemia. He remained speechless as his blue eyes welled up with tears: I knew that he was thinking all the other parents in this room had hoped the same thing for their children, too.

The doctor came back two hours later. "It's not leukemia," he said. "It's a reactive marrow, indicating that his body is reacting to some other process that is producing these symptoms."

Although thrilled with this news, we still did not know what was wrong with him. In the following weeks, we saw specialist after specialist. A joint specialist removed fluid from the left ankle on two occasions and sent it for every diagnostic test possible, including one for Lyme disease. (I had told the doctors that my wife found a small tick on Eric four months earlier while in the Connecticut countryside.) Every test, however, was inconclusive, and the doctors were all stumped. I asked whether Eric could have Lyme disease even with four negative blood tests. They all felt that since the blood tests were done at several different labs, we should rely on them. Yet I felt, both deep in my heart and with my mind, that it made sense to treat Eric for Lyme disease—even without the confirmation of a joint fluid test or a blood test. The rheumatologist and the infectious disease specialist were both against this approach. However, he was my son, and I knew I had to trust my intuition.

Five days after the medication was started, Eric's limp completely disappeared. Ten days after, the rheumatologist could find no evidence of swelling in the ankle. Repeat blood tests were all normal within two weeks. Eric has been healthy ever since. I am certain in retrospect that Eric had Lyme arthritis, which, although it was impossible to prove definitely, was cured with twenty dollars' worth of amoxicillin.

I realized that key to this experience was furthering my *own* healing, as well as that of my wife and son, by learning to trust my inner sense.

3

An Ancient Basis for Modern Medicine

Many doctors are already aware of the role of stress, emotional trauma, improper diet, pessimism, and depression as contributing factors in disease. Many want to learn about forms of treatment such as acupuncture and nutrition. The movement of medicine back toward its original intention to heal has already begun, as physicians have opened their minds to ideas, new and old. But now they must take the next step—making society aware of the need for healing on all levels. They must become aware not only of the great responsibility that has been bestowed on them but also of their own power to heal, waiting to be unleashed.

THE DOCTOR–PATIENT RELATIONSHIP

Hippocrates said, "Some patients, though conscious that their condition is perilous, recover their health simply through their contentment with the goodness of the physician." Sadly, however, this sort of doctor–patient relationship is becoming harder and harder to find. Many patients tell me they feel trapped in their relationship with a doctor or medical center, but they are often unsure why. I always ask them if they feel kindness is radiating from the one providing their care. If the answer to this question is no, then we need to ask what other foundation a healing relationship can possibly be built on. I have heard the Dalai Lama, the spiritual leader of Tibet, ask why kindness could not be one of the world's great religions. By the same token, kindness could be the world's best medicine. Kindness is the essential element if a healing bond is to occur. I do not believe a healing relationship can be built only on chemotherapy, radiation therapy, or reputation.

Of course, I know very well the demands placed on physicians. In addition to helping patients who are in pain, and comforting spouses and children, doctors must make hundreds of complex choices daily. There are the constant inquiries from insurance companies asking for justification of medical decisions that any second-year medical student could make, and the daily calls from "managed-care coordinators" who ask continually when a patient undergoing a standard two-week course of treatment is going home. With all this, as well as the years of school and training required (twelve years for most subspecialists) and the debts incurred in the process, it isn't any wonder that doctors are under constant stress or believe that their position warrants significant financial compensation.

Ultimately, doctors feel that getting too close to the pain they have pledged to alleviate will jeopardize the control they have over their practices and their lives. With all the dilemmas they face, the only option seems to be to close themselves off and protect their privacy. But when physicians attempt to avoid their patients' pain and try to separate themselves from it, they become detached. And this detachment leads to an isolation that the patients see simply as noncaring.

Believe it or not, all doctors would like to say, "I understand and I reach out to you with compassion." But it is one thing to reach out with love and compassion to one patient or family, and quite another to have the energy and reserve to do so for hundreds. When a doctor seems aloof, patients feel he or she no longer has the ability to understand what they are going through or what is in their heart. The doctor, in turn, feels saddened by the fact that patients no longer give him or her the respect and reverence doctors of prior generations knew.

WHAT WE EXPECT AND DEMAND FROM OUR DOCTORS

As a society, we Americans have come to expect "results." Unconsciously, we've decided that death has become an option technology can not only put off but actually save us from. We look at sickness and dying as ultimate failures. We want, and feel we deserve, success, which includes health and a long life. We have incorporated this philosophy into public policy, and to protect ourselves from failure—illness, poverty, death—we remove it from our sight. We put our old people in nursing homes, our poor and homeless in shelters, and our dying in hospices.

A society that values "success" above all else has little room for caring, healing relationships. And if doctors want to reestablish their role as healers, they must realize that when they wall themselves off from their patients, they cannot discover the deeper meaning and purpose of their profession. By giving in to frustration or by escaping into separation, doctors are missing the compassion and joy of imparting healing and the ability to open their hearts to their patients.

Doctors think that patients ask too much. Patients think that doctors provide too little. Everyone thinks medicine has become too expensive, too technical, and too bureaucratic—you don't need a degree in economics to know that the medical system is in crisis. Spiraling insurance premiums, escalating hospital fees, the exorbitant cost of drugs, a federal bureaucracy that denies preventive and diagnostic care to low-income families and the elderly, the politicization of health issues, and the scarcity of doctors in rural areas —all are symptoms of a breakdown in the compact between patients and doctors.

As public frustration intensifies, patients grow more and more unrealistic in their demands. They assume that expensive technology can solve all their problems. They expect doctors to perform miracles with CAT scans, magnetic resonance imaging (MRI) machines, wonder drugs, and space-age hospital intensive care units (ICUs). On the other hand, doctors—frustrated by an overtaxed Medicare system, skyrocketing costs of malpractice insurance, and excessive regulations—cannot attend fully to their patients' needs. To provide the "results" patients expect, doctors order even more diagnostic tests, change medications, and make referrals to subspecialists. This system of "supply-side" health care, which alienates patients and physicians, blocks the relationship that needs to exist for healing to occur.

WHAT WE REALLY WANT AND NEED FROM OUR DOCTORS

Healing is what patients want when they go to their doctors, and healing is what desperately needs to be restored to the medical profession. Healing of illness, healing of suffering, healing of doctors, and healing of patients—this is the truth we need in place of all our solutions. This truth—that healing in its broadest sense is what we are looking for—is in our hearts, where there are no limits to giving and compassion.

We must also have the wisdom to find perspective in our lives. Doctors need to have a sense of perspective that will enable them to open their hearts without feeling drained or diminished. All of us need to stop looking to technology and bureaucracies to save us from discomfort. If we insist on separating ourselves from our essence in such a way, we will continue to live in a state of emotional and spiritual contraction, looking for healing only outside ourselves and finding only disappointment in the medical profession.

Michael: Cancer and Dreams

■ I saw Michael when I was a resident in internal medicine, long before I developed the ESSENCE process. He was eighteen years old, and his cancer of the thymus gland had spread widely. He told me of a recurring dream that he had been having months before he became ill.

"I am on a rafting trip with my class," he recalled. "We start out crossing a narrow point in the river on foot, carrying the rafts to the other side by crossing on some rocks. The rest of the class crosses without a problem, but I fall and am swept away in the river, out to the ocean to drown." This dream foretold Michael's fate.

Michael had just graduated from high school and was preparing to leave home. He was crossing from one threshold in his life to another, and the dream symbolically reflected this crossing. But being swept away while his classmates survived the passage indicated that he was not going to make this transition. The ocean is often symbolic of death, and his being swept to it by way of the river implied death was close at hand. While Michael responded initially to chemotherapy, all his responses to increasingly aggressive regimens were only transient. He died five months later.

Obviously, most dreams about death don't imply that death is imminent. But recurrent dreams often signify that a transformation is occurring, or that an emotion or other part of us for which we have no further use in our lives needs to be discarded. I believe that dreams may provide a window into the depths of what lies within one's soul, and attention to them provides a valuable tool in discovering important issues that a patient may not be aware of consciously. Dream interpretation is thus an important part of the ESSENCE process.

When an unwanted event takes us by surprise, we tend to say it is simply bad luck. This kind of denial releases us from responsibility, but it also leaves us largely powerless. If, however, we look into the origin of illness and ask what purpose it serves or what message it may convey, we become empowered to find healing, because we know where to look for it. To prevent and cure illness, doctors and patients must include the realm of the unconscious mind and the soul in their search for healing. But such an exploration of the mind and soul cannot take place without an atmosphere of trust.

TRUST: THE BASIS FOR HEALING

How do our unconscious minds, emotions, and traumatic experiences influence health and contribute to illness? Fritz Perls, a pioneer of Gestalt psychology (a school of thought that emphasizes people's perception of wholeness), described the process of *assimilation* in personality development. Perls proposed that our repressed memories and painful past experiences in their "unassimilated" state weaken and drain our health. He likened the assimilation process to chewing food. The undigested parts always return in an annoying, distasteful way to cause hardship or illness for the person. He saw that, when ignored, emotions, painful experiences, and conflicts drain our energy and eventually return in the form of depression or illness. Perls wrote that awareness of, and ability to endure, unwanted emotions is necessary for a cure.

If we have *illusions* of peace, security, and health, these are at the expense of our inner being. Many of us have traded our inherent optimism and joy for the delusions of success and achievement taught to us by our parents, teachers, and peers. We have given up our freedom, creativity, and love so we can buy into a Hollywood vision of a successful life that is impossible to attain. We sacrifice our creativity for what we believe is a good education, but what is instead a deceptive view of security and happiness. The results are stressful jobs, a daily struggle for survival, and a level of frustration that is the result of greed and ambition.

As the psychiatrist R. D. Laing noted in *The Divided Self*: "Our 'normal, adjusted' state is too often the abdication of ecstasy, the betrayal of our true potentialities. . . . Many of us are only too successful in acquiring a false self to adapt to false realities." And love, we learn, is to be given only to those who give it back to us.

EMPOWERING THE PATIENT

The most constructive doctor–patient relationship is one that fosters mutual trust and empowers the patient (and often the doctor) to look inward at his or her essence. Though they may be unaware of it at first, most patients yearn for this kind of interaction. That is why I urge my patients to write about their dreams, talk with me about what has been going on in their lives, and practice ESSENCE Guided Imagery meditations. At the very least, meditation and dream awareness can be powerful openings to self-knowledge and spiritual awakening. Without a spiritual component, healing is incomplete.

As a physician, I was taught that my basic goal was to alleviate suffering. But the ancient Chinese text called the *Tao Te Ching* says about the physician: "He brings men back to what they have lost. He helps the ten thousand things find their own nature, but refrains from action." So I have come to realize that there is more to focus on than eliminating symptoms. Physicians must begin to see that when the light of a patient's essence shines on a symptom—whether it be anxiety, depression, or illness—the symptom lessens. For true healing to occur, the well-intentioned desire simply to eliminate suffering must be combined with wisdom.

Illness sometimes allows us to acquire a measure of that wisdom by enabling us to acknowledge a part of ourselves we have not been aware of. If we listen to the messages that an illness may convey, we learn about ourselves and take a major step in regaining our health. In the face of adversity or illness, suddenly the daily diversions, familiar routines, and comfortable illusions cease to be of value. At that point, the yearning to discover the truth of who we really are begins to be aroused. This yearning may be heard clearly, if we will only listen. Illness can thus help lead us to an awareness of our essence and can be a catalyst to personal transformation.

Most patients who are ill have a yearning—conscious or unconscious—to embark on this journey. Often this yearning is so completely repressed that it takes a great deal of talking and counseling before they even become aware of it. So an environment of trust and safety must be created for a doctor to assist patients on this healing journey and provide them with a forgiving, nonjudgmental relationship that extends beyond fear and illness. Trust allows this relationship to develop with mutual benefit to patient and physician. The doctor and patient become true healers together.

4

Learning about Healing

As a medical student, I was made to feel that I was entering a great tradition. In one sense, this tradition stretched back to the ancient Greeks Hippocrates and Galen. But in a much more practical sense, it began less than 150 years ago, with the discoveries of the French chemist Louis Pasteur. He found that microorganisms can be destroyed by heat and that vaccines can be made from weakened strains of some disease-causing microorganisms. Among other things, he "pasteurized" milk and developed a human rabies vaccine from the saliva of a rabid dog.

The German bacteriologist Robert Koch followed Pasteur by learning how to grow cultures of microorganisms and use them medically. The English surgeon Joseph Lister used carbolic acid as an antiseptic, and thus dramatically reduced the incidence of postoperative infections.

With these and other developments, people began to look on medicine as one of the new wonders of the modern world, which indeed it was. Disease was seen to be caused by outside microbes that invaded the body. All doctors had to do, it seemed, was kill the microbes and thereby kill the diseases. For heavily populated parts of Europe, where people died in huge numbers from regular epidemics, this was the promise of a new era. The link between dirt, putrefaction, and disease became understood, and the concept of what we call public health became widespread. Sources of drinking water were protected, sewers were improved, and people began washing their hands with soap before eating. It was seen as only a matter of time, money, and ingenuity before humankind conquered disease. This view spread even more after the medical and scientific necessities of World War II set in motion the new wave of discovery and invention that continues today.

GOING BEYOND SCIENTIFIC DISCOVERY

The most up-to-date knowledge, medication, and instruments *do* make all kinds of medically wonderful things happen. I depend on them in my practice, as every other competent medical specialist does. But I would go so far as to say that not many of us in the developed world today fully comprehend how much suffering has been alleviated by the medical revolution that began with Pasteur. We cannot understand because we ourselves have not had to go through what past generations did: we have been spared by science.

My fellow medical students and I had every reason to believe that we also would do our bit to advance this medical revolution any way we could and bring its benefits to everyone we could. My guess is that the vast majority of us have done so. On the other hand, I could also guess that most of us have found real patients to be far more complex than the textbooks suggested. For example, even if the cause of a person's disease was a simple invasion of microbes from outside the body, we have to wonder why the attack occurred. We have to ask why one person has succumbed to the invasion, while others have resisted it. And we have to try to answer why one person recovered and another died in similar circumstances.

During my hospital internship and my first years as a qualified physician, I was intensely busy familiarizing myself with symptoms, procedures, medications, and so on. I had neither the time nor the inclination to question what I had been taught. Only when I grew more certain of my abilities and gained the power to control my schedule better, could I follow up on some of the unexplainable recoveries that intrigued me.

DISCOVERING THE LINK BETWEEN
CANCER AND PERSONALITY

To keep up with the latest medical findings, I, like other doctors, have to read constantly. I once came across several references in journals to an observation that the psychologist Eugene Blumberg had made in the 1950s regarding cancer incidence. Intrigued, I looked up Blumberg's own reports of his work at a veterans' hospital in Long Beach, California. Blumberg had noticed that personality type seemed to have a lot to do with how fast a patient's cancer progressed and how well that patient responded to therapy. To confirm this, he had given the patients psychological tests to measure their stress and depression levels, and their ability to release tension. Patients who were overcooperative, overnice, overanxious, painfully sensitive, passive, and apologetic usually had the most rapidly progressing disease. In contrast, patients with more expressive and sometimes bizarre personalities usually responded excellently to therapy, had remissions, and survived for longer times.

"You're right!" I shouted (which got me a few curious looks around the medical library), for I had noticed this on the wards myself, but I had been trained to regard such things as outside the concerns of medicine. Things to do with personality were supposed to belong to psychiatry, and I had chosen cancer treatment as my specialty.

One patient of Blumberg's particularly struck me. Diagnosed with breast cancer, she had refused medical treatment on religious grounds, saying her belief gave her all the strength she needed. Ten years later, she still survived. This was something I had yet to see. Nonetheless, while a student, I might have dismissed her case with some rationalization or scientific question. Now that I was a doctor and had seen something of real life and real sickness, I was not so sure. Blumberg's conclusion was that those patients who had found a way to deal with stress had also found a way to resist or at least slow down cancer. He did not know how they did this, but as a responsible healer always does, he let others know who might be able to put his suggestion to use.

Other healers have made similar but independent observations. Elida Evans, a student of Carl Jung, was one of the first people to notice a connection between personality and cancer. In *The Psychological Study of Cancer*, published in 1926, she noted that the kind of people who developed cancer were those whose life's meaning came from other people, jobs, or other things outside themselves. She wrote: "Cancer is a symbol, as most illness is, of something going wrong in the patient's life, a warning to him to take another road."

The New York psychiatrist Lawrence LeShan and his co-workers compared the life stories of 250 cancer patients with those of people hospitalized for other disorders. The lives of the cancer patients were unusually similar to one another and different from those of the other patients. Most had had a lonely childhood, and their unhappy relationships with one or both parents affected their view of later relationships with others. He, too, found that there were people who, as adults, tended to build their life around a cause, an occupation, or a person. When their life purpose fell apart, they became deeply depressed and were found to have cancer less than a year later. At Jefferson Medical College in Philadelphia, the psychologist Claus Bahnson found that cancer patients very often suppressed their emotions and had cold, aloof parents. And British researcher David Kissen also noticed that Scottish lung cancer patients seemed to be emotionally detached from their parents and siblings, and they kept their relatively few emotions about other things pent up.

HEALERS AND SCIENTISTS

Observations about links between cancer and personality are very difficult to prove scientifically, because scientists demand that they themselves be able to repeat the experiment and achieve the same result before they accept a discovery. While this approach works well with experiments in glass test tubes or with fast-breeding generations of fruit flies, it works less well with long-lived higher animals—and it doesn't work at all with humans. Unlike guinea pigs, people cannot be watched constantly or confined beyond reasonable bounds, and their health or life cannot be jeopardized for the sake of a research result. Furthermore, they can't always be believed! Lab rats don't lie, but people often have highly subjective versions of what happens to them. So when scientists apply their strict standards to observations based on what people say, they often have no option but to shoot down the claims because there can be so much variation. In doing this, the scientists are not necessarily unfeeling robots in white coats. They are simply trying to maintain the integrity of research.

The mistake lies in submitting healing phenomena to standards that were not designed to measure them in the first place. This confuses medicine with hard science, and the result is that physical things that can be scientifically observed are considered inherently more meaningful to our health than things that cannot be so recorded. However, this doesn't take into consideration healing's own equally rigorous standard, which is that a thing either helps or doesn't help. Differing responses among individuals will often leave room for some uncertainty, but if something works for seven out of ten people—such as the new antidepressants like Prozac—that's wonderful news for healers, who look at the seven people *helped* and are delighted. Hard scientists, on the other hand, look at the three people who are not helped and decide that more research is needed. While they are almost invariably right, the seven people who can benefit should not be deprived of something in the meantime that can relieve their suffering.

I am not suggesting that medical research be carried out under less stringent safeguards than other forms of scientific research, and a hard-science approach to healing can be rewarding. I ask only that the limitations of hard science not be imposed without justification on the art of healing.

As a matter of fact, a hard-science study published in the British journal *Lancet* in 1989 opened up American physicians' eyes to the reality of something beyond mechanical science being involved in medicine. With colleagues at Stanford University and the University of California at Berkeley, psychiatrist David Spiegel had set out to test scientifically whether there was anything to these stories about a tie between stress and the rapid progression of cancer. He fully expected to find none.

The study involved stress counseling for women with advanced breast cancer. The women were selected randomly. One group was counseled for stress, and the other was not. Allowances were made for various factors that might affect the results. The women who received counseling for stress had a median survival time of 36.6 months, and those who did not receive counseling had a median survival time of 18.9 months.

These were results that even skeptics could duplicate. To date, no one has disputed Dr. Spiegel's startling results. A small but significant percentage increase in survival for the counseled women would have pleased those already convinced that stress plays a role in disease, but none would have dared make the claim that counseling for stress can double the life expectancy of a woman with advanced breast cancer. Yet this study justified such a claim.

STRESS AND ESSENCE
GUIDED IMAGERY

Like many other health care professionals, I became convinced of the dangers of stress a decade before Dr. Spiegel's paper was published. Our chief concern as healers was not getting scientific proof of what we observed in our patients but finding some way to neutralize stress's damaging effects. However, the relationship between stress and disease is not a simple cause-and-effect one. Stress does not seem to cause disease *directly;* it works more circuitously, perhaps by helping to trigger risk factors or suppress the immune system. We still do not know for sure.

Much has been written in recent years about stress and its role in health, and attitudes have greatly changed—superficially at least. But in the actual practice of medicine, things have been slower to change, and some things have not changed at all. This fact is what prompted me to develop the ESSENCE program.

5

Science and Mind/Body Health

The ESSENCE program will help you manage stress. It enables you to put sufficient spiritual space between your higher self and the event that is causing you distress. This space permits you to be resilient and to *manage* what stress is doing to you, rather than being a puppet whose strings are constantly pulled this way and that.

STRESS AND THE BODY

It is now rare to find a newstand magazine article on health that doesn't mention the damaging effects of stress. Stress has been implicated in the onset, course, and outcome of many physical and mental illnesses. Some people even claim it is the major killer of our time. The relationship between stress and illness, however, is more complex than some writers suggest. To protect ourselves, we need to understand first what happens in our bodies under stressful conditions.

The word *stress* has taken on many meanings in both popular and scientific accounts. Some people use the word to refer to an event or stimulus outside us that causes discomfort. Others use the word to refer to the actual discomfort we feel. To add to the confusion, some people also use the word interchangeably. To define the phenomenon of stress more precisely, many researchers use other words to describe what is involved. They may call the event or stimulus outside the person the *stressor*. The stressor causes *distress* in the person. And the distress leads to a *consequence,* which may involve illness. Things that affect any of these three stages may be called *mediators.* The following diagram may help show this more clearly.

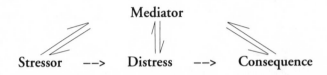

Stressor   -->   Distress   -->   Consequence

Viewing stress as having separate components helps us understand it as a multistep process instead of a simple stimulus and reaction. But thinking of stress in these terms may seem to suggest that every stressor elicits distress. Not all stressful events, however, produce a stress response, for the likelihood of producing such a response depends on many psychological and biological factors, and these factors may also act as mediators. For example, a stressful event for someone with a normal heart may produce only a rapid heartbeat, whereas for someone who has coronary heart disease, the same event may lead to anginal pain or even heart failure. Similarly, a family history of high blood pressure increases the likelihood that an individual will react to a stressful event with a response involving the cardiovascular system. Personality, behavior, social factors, age, gender, ethnicity, and economic status may all act as mediators in the stressor-distress process. Rather than look for a single cause of stress and its effect on our health, we need to consider all the personal and environmental factors that may be involved.

Stressors cause both mental and physical changes in our bodies. This happens because of the links between our brain and our cardiovascular, gastrointestinal, and other body systems—including even our immune system.

THE HPA AXIS AND OUR HEALTH

In general, researchers today hold that the brain has two major routes for communication with the body: the hypothalamic-pituitary-adrenal (HPA) axis and the involuntary nervous system.

Stressors are perceived in the brain, and signals are sent to the hypothalamus, a part of the brain that regulates many functions of the body. When the hypothalamus receives signals prompted by exposure to a stressful event, it secretes something called cortisol releasing hormone (CRH). This is then carried within the brain by the blood to the pituitary gland, which is frequently referred to as the "master gland," since it regulates the whole endocrine, or hormone, system, including the adrenal cortex, thyroid gland, ovaries, and testes. When CRH stimulates the pituitary, adrenocorticotropic hormone (ACTH) is released into the bloodstream. This in turn triggers the adrenal cortex to secrete corticosteroid hormones, such as cortisol.

The hormone cortisol powerfully affects the body's metabolism of proteins, carbohydrates, and fats. It breaks down proteins in the tissues, releasing amino acids into the bloodstream that can then be used to repair injured tissues. Cortisol also helps convert amino acids into carbohydates that can then be broken down for energy, and it converts fats to energy. Cortisol can increase twentyfold in the blood in response to stressors.

Corticosteroid hormones, or corticosteroids, control cardiovascular functions and suppress inflammation. They are therefore essential for many of the body functions necessary for adaptation to stressors—in other words, the body's means of dealing with stress. An overreaction of ACTH, however, can have an adverse effect and can lead to such conditions as high blood pressure or diabetes, or to suppression of the immune system. But, fortunately, we have a built-in regulatory system that works much like a thermostat. Just as the heat is turned off by the thermostat when the temperature rises above a set point, activity of the HPA system is inhibited in the hypothalamus and pituitary when the level of corticosteroids in the bloodstream increases. This built-in feedback system pro-brain is so actively involved in our stress responses, it is only logical that our reactions to stressful events should be reflected in our behavior. For some people, stressful experiences may be of such a nature or intensity that they lead to the onset of serious mental disorders, such as depression and panic attacks.

For most of us, the reaction is less severe: we may feel keyed up, tense, or frightened in stressful situations. But our thinking may be influenced by these situations, and, at times, we may become confused. Stressors may also lead to maladaptive actions such as increased smoking, overconsumption of alchol, or drug abuse. However, as with bodily responses to stressors, behavioral reactions are specific to individuals: events that lead to behavioral changes for one person may not do the same for another, and mediators often influence the outcome.

DON'T OVERSIMPLIFY

It would be unrealistically simplistic to expect, in our complicated lives, that our stress arises from a single stressor producing distress and resulting in a single consequence. Several stress processes are likely to be in operation at any given time, and they may or may not be linked with or dependent on one another. In addition, within a single stress process, stressors may be multiple and either independent or linked. So, too, may be the consequences. To regard all stress as bad is another oversimplification. Many people learn to use pressure as a goad to achievement.

Although we vary greatly as individuals in our reactions to specific things, we tend to be helped or harmed in similar ways. What's good for one person may be even better for another, but only rarely will it be bad for someone. Conversely, what's bad for one person may not be so harmful for another, but only rarely will it be good for anyone. Although we are complex and we vary, we can each learn to manage our individual level of stress in our own personal way from ESSENCE healing.

Stress, of course, is as much a part of the mind as of the body.

We now look briefly at what psychiatrists and psychologists have discovered.

THE SCIENCE OF THE MIND

It's not as if modern medicine has ignored the mind. However, the treatment of mental and emotional disorders has been compartmentalized, neatly labeled "psychiatry and psychology," and put on a shelf. Physicians tend not to reach for anything on that shelf until they have tried just about everything else on other shelves.

Doctors trained to diagnose physical symptoms naturally look for physical signs of illness. When they do not find what they are looking for, they look harder and consider the possibility of a rare disease. Only when they have exhausted the possibility of every physical cause of illness do they consider an emotional cause, and even then they are likely to hesitate before calling in a psychiatrist or psychologist.

There are several good reasons for this approach. First, doctors see it as an admission of failure. Second, they know that many patients would react negatively to a referral and would take this to mean that they're seen as crazy. But this referral gap between regular physicians and psychiatrists and psychologists is unfortunate, because the latter can amplify the diagnoses of the former in ways that help the patient. Although psychiatrists are trained in the same tradition as other physicians, they often have a much less conventional view of illness, and they have no trouble in seeing the mental or emotional component in many physical sicknesses. Psychologists, of course, have a training highly focused on the mental and emotional aspects. Within the limits of their discipline, psychiatrists and psychologists claim that healing the inner person can also heal the physical disorder.

Endless classification and reclassification of knowledge is part of the scientific tradition. The American Psychiatric Association has organized and numbered emotional disorders in a system similar to that used for cataloguing library books. The system is published as the *Diagnostic and Statistical Manual of Mental Disorders* (known as the *DSM*) and is used internationally by clinical practitioners.

For example, a patient named Josephine Smith was assigned the *DSM* numbers 307.10, 305.20, and 301.13. Another psychiatrist or psychiatric nurse looking at her medical chart would know from these numbers what to expect from her in general, plus which medications to give her and which to avoid. They would not find her diagnosis of several disorders very unusual, and many would recognize the numbers without having to look them up: anorexia nervosa (307.10), cannabis abuse (305.20), and cyclothymia (301.13), a form of depression. But from these numbers, we still have no idea who Josephine Smith is, or *why* she is this way.

Such a situation is not caused by present-day psychiatrists' or psychologists' lack of empathy for their patients. In urban clinics, large numbers of people seek help from a limited number of professionals and often are treated by different staff members on different visits. Cultural and linguistic differences can also complicate matters. A system such as *DSM* numbering ensures consistency of treatment in such situations. If they know a certain kind of emergency exists, psychiatrists can try to stabilize patients with medication and advice, so they do not hurt themselves or others. However, once the patients are stabilized temporarily, they often drop out of sight, and the psychiatrists never see them again.

These realities of urban medicine are not the doctors' fault. Many psychiatrists and psychologists spend grueling, thankless hours trying to help people whom society has cast aside as unwanted. Most are hard-working physicians and therapists who struggle against lack of understanding and the emotional distress engendered in people by our complex and fast-changing society. Just as I would insist that a person with a tumor see an oncologist, I would insist that a person with a mental or emotional disorder seek help from a psychiatrist or psychologist.

The *DSM* avoids defining exactly what a mental disorder is. The book uses the yardstick that if your problem is big enough to interfere with your daily functioning, it qualifies as a mental disorder. Things with everyday causes, such as a dispute with your landlord, do not qualify. As a result, most of us don't have a mental or emotional disorder as defined by psychiatrists. For anything beneath the level of a classifiable disorder, the labeling system is vague: what might be seen as a mild depression by one person could be seen by another as a spiritual malaise. But there's an important difference between these two viewpoints. Saying that someone has a mild depression implies little or no responsibility on the person's part. On the other hand, if you say someone has a spiritual malaise, you may be suggesting that a character flaw is involved. And while blame may be just the thing to rouse some people out of a spiritual malaise, it is equally likely to make others sink farther into their depression.

Physicians cannot set themselves up as moral guardians. They usually have had varied experiences with people and know that their own personal code of behavior can easily be misunderstood by others with a different background. Psychiatry and psychology were never meant to—nor do they—provide us with answers to spiritual questions. Nevertheless, healers of all kinds have much to learn from the insights of modern psychiatrists and psychologists.

SOMATIZATION

Of particular interest to me, in my search for things relevant to the inner healing power, has been the phenomenon of somatization. The New York psychiatrist Berney Goodman, in his book *When the Body Speaks Its Mind,* defines *somatization* as the way people express emotional discomfort through physical symptoms rather than words. For example, you may develop a tension headache at the prospect of having to entertain one of your spouse's business associates. Once the event is over, your headache disappears. Another example is lower back pain after a stressful day of office work. A warm bath, a good meal, or an amusing TV program usually provides the distraction and relaxation to make the backache go away. This is perfectly normal. According to Dr.

Goodman, 60 to 80 percent of Americans have at least one somatization symptom per week, and most of us are more likely to express our emotional discomfort through physical symptoms than through words. We are communicating our feelings, even if we don't know it.

Somatization should not be confused with psychosomatic illness, such as a duodenal ulcer or ulcerative colitis, where a real physical illness is present. In somatization, there is no physical illness. However, if we begin imagining that these somatization symptoms have a medical cause, we start to become hypochondriacs. Such hypochondria is not as rare as you might think: in a study done more than a decade ago, researchers found that American doctors were billing patients for $20 billion per year for somatization symptoms—about 10 percent of U.S. health costs at that time.

DEPRESSION

While it's true that when we are sick we are more likely to be depressed, it also seems to be true that we are more likely to become sick when we are depressed. Depression may contribute to our *vulnerability* to illness, and it may interact with stress in unknown ways.

The *DSM* classifies depression into a number of mood disorders. The so-called milder forms of depression, such as prolonged mourning, the "blues," sadness, and constant tiredness, are not included in these clinical mood disorders. These are some of the emotional states that can most readily be alleviated by our inner healing power through the use of spiritual techniques.

INNER LIFE

I purposely left out the words *spiritual* and *religious* from this section's heading because I knew that many people would see those words only as warning flags to skip ahead. Speaking as someone who understands this reaction very well, let me deal with it directly and briefly.

Many feel, justifiably, that as young people, their spiritual inclinations were repressed or damaged by the authoritarianism and rigidity of clergy or self-appointed moral guardians. They point out, correctly, that being religious does not in itself mean having a personal spiritual life. In fact, some believe there might be more spirituality around if there were less organized religion.

As I mentioned in the foreword, my ESSENCE program does not involve religious belief. However, it very much involves a spiritual life. The amount your religious belief helps or hinders your spiritual life is therefore the amount it affects your ESSENCE program.

Many of us were fortunate enough to have had early teachers or families who used religion as a tried-and-true path to spiritual life. Such people do not have to be persuaded that, in a time of trial, their belief and spiritual power have helped them survive and recover from things that would otherwise have finished them. This is something they know from experience. They would smile if you asked them to prove it scientifically.

We all know what religions are. Each involves a more or less fixed set of beliefs, the major ones of which you have to accept or appear to accept in order to belong. It's much harder to define *spiritual life*. The clergy use religious terms to describe it. Psychiatrists may diagnose it as a symptom of an emotional disorder. Both classical composers and jazz musicians have tried to convey it through the sound of their instruments.

Spiritual life has traditionally been seen as a journey or quest. The goal is often cloaked in mystery or ambiguity, but the striving to achieve it is what counts. This striving typically tests us, requiring that we fall back on our resources and use all our talents and capabilities. Most of us, of course, settle for a less arduous course—but the ideal is there.

A comfortable life is not very conducive to spiritual quests. Very often it is only when something strongly interferes with our comforts that we resort to our spiritual side. And that intruder is frequently illness.

Spiritual power and religious belief help us bear sorrow and stress. In poor health, they promote recovery and prolong survival. In good health, they help us enjoy a harmonious life and handle unavoidable stress, and they even build resilience in those who thrive on stress and excitement.

Long before there were physicians, humans knew they had an inner healing force or power. Different cultures have approached it in different ways, but all tap into the same source. A modern American doctor, in our multicultural society, has to try to be all things to all people. But, like everyone else, doctors are limited by their own personalities, background, and education. So, however, are their patients! This sometimes leads to communication problems on even the simplest levels. When it comes to discussing an invisible healing power within ourselves—something that we all have and that only needs to be released—we must first create an atmosphere of openness and trust.

I am a doctor, a scientist, a healer—not a theologian or a philosopher. I respect those who are, and I do not see medicine as being beyond the bounds of religion, ethics, or scientific principles. I speak always from the point of view of healing. If something heals and at the same time cannot be understood by the intellect, we have to be willing to look beyond the intellectual mind.

To avoid as many communication problems as I can—and also, I admit, to gloss over things I do not know—I use the word *essence* in the sense that I first heard it when I was twelve. I usually feel a little hesitant about first mentioning essence to a patient in a consulting room in Manhattan, often with the latest biotechnological instruments purring and blinking nearby. And I know our old family friend Dominguez would only smile.

The meditations and spiritual paths of the ESSENCE process can guide and protect us in our seemingly indifferent, impersonal, overly material, high-tech world. Throughout history, essence is all that humans have ever had to allay their fears of a hostile environment. We have always depended on our higher self for physical survival, knowing that without survival of the spirit, hostile elements would triumph.

Part Two

THE
ESSENCE
GUIDED
IMAGERY
PROCESS

6

Introduction to the ESSENCE *Guided Imagery Process*

Nature and God—I neither knew
Yet Both so well knew me
They startled, like Executors
Of My identity.
—*Emily Dickinson,* No. 835, st. 1

Awakening to your essence will reveal not what is right or wrong, but simply *what is.* This awakening requires only that you wake up to your inner light and become aware of its power and beauty. The ESSENCE process is directed at the physical, emotional, and spiritual aspects of each person. Counseling, nutritional support, and medication all have a critical role, as do the guided imagery meditations outlined in this book. But this book is not meant to be a complete guide to the process of awakening to your inner being—and it could not be, because everyone has different needs and experiences.

As long as we are unwilling to receive the truth of our essence, this will be manifest in a symbolic way through our body or mind. We must therefore pay attention to the direction in which a dysfunction or depression is trying to lead us. The more we resist, deny, or try to relieve the symptom, the more dysfunction we will develop.

ESSENCE healing allows us to accept our illness or adversity so that we can use it to bring out wisdom, light, and truth from our soul. This healing brings about an experience of the reality of our essence. It also brings us guidance, which may bring us the wisdom that our essence intended for us to learn through illness. Enlightened people are willing to surrender to their hearts to learn the truth of their essence. Healing done with this intent will always attract the intended guidance.

The ESSENCE process allows us to heal our fear. Many of us live in a constant state of fear that has been so persistent we are no longer even aware of it. Some of us do not really understand that free will is inherent in life and that all things are possible— illness and health, love and hate, violence and kindness. ESSENCE Guided Imagery requires only an *open mind*—not discipline, practice, or concentration. We need not have an image of what healing should feel like or what should be its end result; this would engender only more fear. The mind can create for us only judgments and resistance; it cannot create truth. Truth comes in periods of silence. Creation of this silence is the beginning of healing. ESSENCE healing leads to a silence that requires almost no effort to create.

To receive the truth of your higher self through the ESSENCE process is to experience the power and peace inherent in who you really are. But you can't just grab or buy this experience. It's an illusion to believe that effort, ambition, and struggle can bring you anything other than money and success. With money and success, you can live a long life without ever knowing a minute of true joy or happiness. The joy and love that flow from your heart when the struggle ceases reveals the simple truth that has been within you all along.

We have most likely been conditioned as to what healing should be and what it should bring about. We think it should produce a result. We think it should be direct and straightforward. To begin the healing paths in this book with those expectations in mind means clinging to old ideas. We have to let go of these expectations about healing, so that it can be experienced free of fear. If we do not free ourselves from being tied down by ideas of what healing should be, we will always cling to the notion that healing must occur in a certain way for a certain end. By confining thoughts of healing to a particular pattern, our mind diminishes the possibilities of healing. We need to let go of what we think healing should be and allow our mind to be still, innocent, and fresh. This way, the miracles of healing can occur. The essence in each of us knows that these miracles are simply its birthright.

Meditation has been described in the literature of the East and West for thousands of years. There are hundreds of different methods and systems, and new schools are developing regularly. Most kinds of meditation involve either concentrating, sitting in a certain posture, practicing breathing, or repeating a mantra (that is, a special or sacred word). However, the meditation described in this book, which can lead you to knowing the truth of your essence, is not done like that.

Meditation that can be of value in knowing your essence requires you to be alert and aware of your thoughts and feelings without judgment or resistance. When you can watch the movement of your thoughts and feelings without judging and resisting them, you will achieve a new type of silence. You will feel the origin of your thoughts and feelings. What is required for this type of meditation? First, the sincere intent to experience your essence must exist. Second, you must be free from your own criticism and judgments about any thoughts and feelings that come up.

ESSENCE Guided Imagery and meditation is thus a state of mind that can look at everything without judgment or resistance. This is a great asset in life because it gives you a window to your soul. The healing guidelines I offer are not rigid methods to learn, so you cannot do them incorrectly, or better or worse than anyone else. These meditations allow you to be aware of your fear, hate, and anger as well as your beauty, compassion, and power—all without judgment or resistance.

ESSENCE imagery is a process of expanding your awareness.

You must understand that an honest commitment and readiness to face all aspects of your life are necessary for you to complete this process. To the degree that you hide negative or painful parts of your life from your awareness and are thus unwilling to deal with them, you will not find the courage to find true healing or learn the wonderful truth of who you are. Also, you cannot skip a step in your own path to healing. If healing depends on removing certain fears, misconceptions, or guilt, then you must deal with these first. If you are not willing to face what blocks out the truth of who you are, then creation of healing in that particular area cannot occur.

Healing may occur as the light of our essence touches the darkness of our misconceptions and fear. We must not be impatient and expect a specific result immediately. The German Jewish philosopher Martin Buber wrote:

> Man is like a tree. If you stand in front of a tree and watch it incessantly to see how it grows, and to see how much it has grown, you will see nothing at all. But tend it at all times, prune the runners and keep it free of beetles and worms, and—all in good time—it will come into its growth. It is the same with man: All that is necessary is for him to overcome his obstacles, and he will thrive and grow. But it is not right to examine him hour after hour to see how much has already been added to his stature.

SEVEN STEPS AND FOUR PATHS

The ESSENCE process allows you to discover the richness, beauty, and power of your essence. You need memorize nothing more than the seven key words from which *ESSENCE* comes. Each meditation has the same seven steps. Here is an example:

1. EXPERIENCE

Experience where in your body you feel the judgments you have about your illness. Feel their exact location, size, shape, color, and temperature. Visualize them as energy.

2. SEE

Visualize the light of your essence located above the top of your head. Visualize it as a white, comforting luminous light which emanates from your essence or higher self.

3. SURRENDER

Surrender your judgments to the higher power of your essence by visualizing their energy being released upwards into the light of your essence.

4. EMPOWER

Empower and strengthen this healing by visualizing the white light of your essence flowing from above your head down to the area where you most experience negative judgments.

5. NURTURE

Nurture the idea of a life free from negative judgments. Visualize these judgments as clouds, and imagine them dispersed by the white light of your essence, leaving a clear, bright blue sky.

6. CREATE

Create a space for your higher power to continue to guide you by visualizing a channel through which the light of your essence can continue to flow in and the negativity you are working with can flow out.

7. EMBODY

Embody and externalize this healing by visualizing the light of your essence flowing into each cell of your body.

Of the seven steps of the ESSENCE Guided Imagery meditations, the first three lead to acceptance, and the remaining four assist in transformation. Acceptance and transformation together lead to a healing perspective. This is how the process looks:

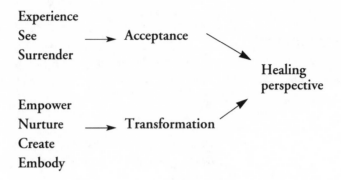

A healing perspective results, first, from accepting whatever adversity or negativity is disturbing us, and allowing this to be transformed by seeing it from the viewpoint of our essence. Problems viewed this way lose much of their destructive energy. Perspective thus provides us with far more calmness and insight than many of the avoidance mechanisms we use to try to escape from the adversities we all must face in life. Avoidance mechanisms such as drugs, alcohol, and overeating only contribute to the negativity in our lives.

I have found that healing on the level of a person's essence is a process or path. Therefore, I have developed four ESSENCE paths that give direction to the meditation. The four ESSENCE paths help us (1) heal fear, (2) go beyond suffering, (3) end melancholy, and (4) create hope. Each healing path is described in its own chapter, followed by a healing meditation to enable you to gain a footing on that path.

These ESSENCE healing paths and meditations are only one of many ways toward healing. All approaches to healing should lead you to the same realization: an awareness of who you really are and of your power to transform your life completely.

LEARNING TO MEDITATE

The ESSENCE Guided Imagery meditations are best done alone in a quiet environment. They may also be done sitting at a table with a pen and paper handy so that you can write down any realizations or lessons that come to you. I recommend that the ESSENCE meditations be done for about twenty minutes, twice daily. The best times are shortly after waking and directly before going to bed at night. Practicing this process will help you develop a skill that will always serve you.

Before beginning any of the ESSENCE Guided Imagery meditations, find a quiet place to sit. If you can, unplug the telephone and be free of any distractions for the twenty-minute period. Sit comfortably on a couch or chair with your eyes closed for two to three minutes. Breathe deeply several times, inhaling into the upper part of your abdomen as fully as you can, then slowly exhaling all the air from your lungs. Concentrate on each breath as you do this. Be conscious of breathing into your stomach by focusing on your abdominal muscles rising and falling. As you do the breathing, with each breath allow yourself to think and feel any of the following positive thoughts with the word *infinite* before them: infinite love, infinite healing, infinite peace, infinite wisdom, infinite harmony, infinite light, infinite hope, and infinite success. (I repeat these instructions later with each meditation.)

UNDERSTANDING WITH THE HEART AND MIND

The ESSENCE Guided Imagery meditations should be done in two stages. Both involve attaining clarity and wisdom—first, on a rational level through your thoughts and, second, on an emotional level through your heart. These are the two fundamental levels through which to attain the necessary wisdom of ESSENCE healing. You understand through your mind by thinking rationally about a concept, seeing how it relates to your life, and then deciding whether or not it makes sense. If it does, you assess it to be true and useful for you.

Understanding through your heart may seem less familiar. To do this, you need to take a concept into your heart on an emotional level and then gauge its truth for you by how it feels. You understand in this way by trying to absorb the concept without judging it, by seeing if you can relate to it on an emotional level. If the concept or idea feels true, you can learn from it. It will be an idea your mind cannot—and was never meant to—understand. This is a part of the process to be experienced, rather than understood with your rational mind.

As a society, we Americans have developed the conceited belief that everything can be rationally understood. The truth is, we can understand only a minute fraction of what we observe in ourselves and our world. This is not to say that we should not try to understand that which can be comprehended. But we should not delude ourselves into thinking we can understand everything. Nor should we waste our time trying to understand with the mind truths we can understand only through the heart.

Francis Bacon, the Elizabethan writer and philosopher, said, "By far the best proof is experience." There is a part of life we can know only by experiencing it, and only by experiencing it can we come to know its validity and power. This experience comes through understanding with the heart. When you can experience certain aspects of your life this way without trying to rationalize them, you will glimpse an important part of life that has, until now, been unknown to you.

ACCEPTANCE OF OURSELVES

The moment we accept ourselves with all our imperfections, we have taken the first step in going beyond ourselves. Our refusal to accept the fear, worry, anger, violence, and greed within ourselves stems from our own denial that we have any of these traits. In this way, we create our ego. In reality, we create a false self whom we pretend to be—a person who is selfless, altruistic, kind, and humble. Carl Jung called the self we disown by accepting only our ideals "the shadow." The ESSENCE process allows you to accept first *all* that is your mind, that which you judge as both good and bad. When you can accept it, you can be transformed. If you can completely accept your entire self, you move to your very essence. Only from this point is transformation and inner healing possible.

But why can't transformation and healing occur at the level of the ego or mind? Well, say that anger is present throughout your life. How will you become less angry? You think to yourself, "I am angry. But from now on I'll no longer allow myself to be an angry person." You picture yourself being without anger—acting compassionately and selflessly. However, this ideal does not actually allow you to truly *accept* that you *are* angry in the first place. An angry ego or mind can never be not-angry. When your angry mind tries to be not-angry, even this effort is being guided by the angry mind. Thus, the mind is only avoiding anger in the very effort to be free of it, creating a false self to cover the anger up and losing the opportunity to accept yourself as you are. And if you never take the first step of *accepting* yourself as you are, you can never take the second step of *discovering* your essence or center, and then *transforming*. In other words, an angry person can learn from his or her anger by accepting it and addressing its cause and purpose, rather than allowing it to assume such importance by constantly battling it. When you stop denying anger, you can begin to let it go.

A person who has been through this process can say, "My mind may always be angry. I have seen my anger and accepted it. Avoiding my anger has hurt me, but when I accepted it, I found I could make use of it without it hurting me. While I need to, I will use my mind's anger to understand lessons I have yet to learn. My mind is only a wall that surrounds my essence: it is not me. When I am centered in my essence, I can make use of that wall rather than be totally identified with it."

Inner healing will never occur when you hold onto the denial and delusions of the ego. You can only be free of your ego when you have truly accepted it, when you can watch it and let it be what it is. This acceptance—free from the ego's judgment or condemnation—brings you to your center, your essence, your higher self. Thus, the first part of the ESSENCE process is to accept, to remain true to yourself. When you can observe your anger, fear, ambition, and greed and accept them, you can see the wall that surrounds your essence, and you can move over it. Then you can begin to transform your life.

7

Releasing Negative Feelings about Illness: Following the Seven Steps

The healing process can have many outcomes. Your ability to release your negative feelings about illness largely depends on how aware of, and aligned with, your essence you can become. The ESSENCE meditations in this book can contribute to this deepening of your awareness. We all have a great deal of confusion about who we are and why we are here. Your commitment and intention to clear this confusion will greatly facilitate healing and health in your life.

The following healing meditation is an example of a seven-step guided imagery meditation. You may also find it useful as an all-purpose meditation—with multiple targets rather than a single one.

ESSENCE
Meditation: Releasing Negative Feelings about Illness

Begin this meditation by sitting on a couch or chair in a quiet place. Take several deep breaths. Slowly inhale, breathing in through your nose and out through your mouth, into your abdomen. Now slowly exhale as completely as you can. Concentrate on each breath. Then simply observe your breathing for another two or three minutes without trying to control it.

As you are taking the deep breaths, visualize a still, deep-blue mountain lake located in the upper part of your abdomen or solar plexus. With each breath repeat to yourself several of the following positive thoughts, with the word *infinite* before each word. For example, think of infinite healing, infinite truth, infinite forgiveness, infinite light, infinite love, infinite peace, or infinite wisdom.

1. EXPERIENCE

Experience your feelings about discomfort or pain and feel how it is affecting your body. Try to localize it and mentally give it a shape, size, temperature, and color. You probably feel that you just want to eliminate the symptoms.

Say to yourself, "I want healing, and for this I must first accept and fully experience how this discomfort is affecting my body."

The rhetorical questions I use in ESSENCE Guided Imagery

are a way of focusing our mind to ask the questions that will lead us to the truth. What questions come up for you? You might ask, "Have I yet experienced my discomfort after really accepting it? Is the way this illness affects my body different than how I have been thinking about it?"

2. SEE

See and behold your higher power or essence. Visualize it as a light above where your awareness is now focused. Visualize your awareness moving into this light.

Say to yourself, "I choose to see and align myself with my higher power, which is real and can never be hurt by discomfort or pain."

Spend several minutes experiencing your illness from the vantage point of your soul, rather than that of your body, which sees only sickness. Be open to any negative thoughts or emotions that come up that may be contributing to the illness.

Be aware of any questions that come forth. You might ask, "Is there a part of me that I can be aware of that has not been affected by this illness? Is there perhaps more of me that has not been hurt than has been?"

3. SURRENDER

Surrender your discomfort or pain to the higher power of your essence.

Say to yourself, "I surrender to my higher power with its infinite compassion, guidance, and wisdom. Whatever healing needs to occur, I will it to occur, with all my power."

For several minutes, contemplate and experience the vast power to heal that this surrender can bring.

Allow any questions to come up. You might ask, "In the context of my essence, what does my illness now feel like? In the context of my essence, what does healing feel like?"

4. EMPOWER

Empower and strengthen this healing by recalling your essence.

Say to yourself, "My pain and suffering are temporary, but I have the power and safety to begin the healing process in this moment."

Your essence does not need words to understand this concept perfectly. Spend several minutes picturing this healing entering every cell of your body—especially the area of discomfort.

5. NURTURE

Nurture and cultivate the idea of the outcome you hope for and would like to be reality—your cure, relief of pain, or whatever you are working on through this meditation.

Say to yourself, "I will cultivate this picture as I would a small tree. I will nurture it daily and help it grow into my physical reality."

In your state of expanded awareness, you do not need to resist what comes up. Spend several minutes imagining the path to this outcome.

Be aware of any questions that come to you. You might ask, "Does the path I'm visualizing feel right for me? Don't I deserve the outcome I'm visualizing?"

6. CREATE

Create a space for your higher power to continue to provide you with appropriate guidance and healing.

Say to yourself, "I have experienced my essence, and while my physical existence has been mostly unaware of this reality, I now surrender to it in total trust to provide healing."

This space you are creating is yours, and you can always return. The more you practice creating it, the easier it will be to return, and the greater will be your power to use it. Spend a few minutes feeling this trust and the energy and power associated with it.

Be aware of any questions that come up. You might ask, "How can my life be different when I am aware of a higher reality and purpose? How do I feel about surrender—even to my own essence?"

7. EMBODY

Embody and externalize this healing. That is, bring the healing into your physical reality and make it a part of your daily life. Visualize the light of your essence flowing into every cell in your body. It is not enough to just visualize this. Allow yourself to feel it.

Say to yourself, "I choose to have what I know I deserve—healing. I choose healing of my spirit, healing of my mind, and healing of my body." This statement will initiate a creative process that will continue to have an effect after this ESSENCE Guided Imagery is over.

Slowly bring your awareness back to your body, which has now been touched by your own healing.

Having done the seven steps with your eyes open, you should do a visualization by performing them with your eyes closed, having familiarized yourself with the text. As a reminder of the seven steps, you may wish to glance at the following box—one appears at the end of each meditation. Remember to do the breathing exercise before starting.

RELEASING NEGATIVE FEELINGS ABOUT ILLNESS: THE SEVEN STEPS WITH YOUR EYES CLOSED

Begin with the breathing exercise.

1. EXPERIENCE

Find the place in your body where you experience negative feelings about discomfort or pain. Feel the exact location of this place and its size, shape, color, and temperature. Visualize all this as energy. Pick only one area of your body at a time.

2. SEE

Visualize the light of your essence located above the top of your head.

3. SURRENDER

Surrender your negative feelings about pain or discomfort to the higher power of your essence by visualizing its energy being released upwards into the light of your essence.

4. EMPOWER

Empower and strengthen this healing by recalling your essence. Feel it as a warm, healing light which you can direct with each in-breath, into the area you are working on.

5. NURTURE

Nurture the idea of a life free of negative judgments.

6. CREATE

Create a space for your higher power to continue to guide you by visualizing a channel through which the light of your essence can continue to flow in and the negativity you are working with can flow out.

7. EMBODY

Embody and externalize this healing by visualizing the light of your essence flowing into each cell of your body.

8

Removing the Barriers to Healing

He who wants to have right without wrong,
Order without disorder,
Does not understand the principles
Of heaven and earth.
He does not know how
Things hang together.
Can a man cling only to heaven
And know nothing of earth?
They are correlative: to know one
Is to know the other.
To refuse one
Is to refuse both.
Can a man cling to the positive
Without any negative
In contrast to which it is seen
To be positive?

—Chuang Tzu

Whenever we experience adversity, our barriers to healing will become apparent. It is during trying times that our separation from our essence becomes so painfully evident. Illness, depression, or loss has the power to bring up guilt and shame that have long been repressed from the conscious mind. These are the very stones that form the wall around our essence. So adversity can actually be an opportunity to rediscover our essence, its truth, and our capacity for healing.

Our need to avoid fear, illness, and suffering rests in our attachment to forgetfulness. When we identify ourselves with who we are not, we avoid everything that would allow us to know who we are. When we are attached to conformity rather than to our uniqueness, to resistance rather than surrender, and to guilt rather than forgiveness, we magnify our pain and intensify our sense of isolation both from others and from our own essence. We will always feel separate from healing to the degree that we feel removed from our essence.

We have become so identified with our thoughts that we think they are all that we are. We thus deny our essence, which exists on some level, without thought. Until we can experience the fact that we are more than our thoughts, more than our bodies with their imperfections, and more than our worries and despairs, we will not be able to let go of the barriers to healing.

Every desire we picture in our mind sets in motion creative processes that work toward its achievement. Once activated by our desires, forces deep in our unconscious begin to attract the people, circumstances, and conditions necessary to actualize what we have pictured. This creative power, whether we realize it or not, has been working either for or against our best interests, depending on the degree to which we have been aware of it. This has been true since we were children. By becoming aware of this process, we can use it to facilitate our transformation and healing.

TRANSFORMATION AND HEALING

Transformation is the path of discovering our essence, and no one can make this discovery for us. This discovery leads to closer relationships with other people and the world. The laws that govern the universe and our lives are impartial and operate continually.

When we live our lives separate from and unaware of our essence, we suffer the consequences of illness, depression, and other maladies in direct proportion to our lack of awareness. When we develop this awareness, we align ourselves with these laws. We benefit to the degree that we can become attuned to this reality.

When we are aware of our higher self and the laws that govern the universe, we no longer act out of fear. We see that to harm another through violence will never bring us protection, but only more violence. We know that to avoid or escape situations and people that we fear will only cause more fear. This truth is contained in a prayer of Saint Francis of Assisi (the thirteenth-century Italian who founded the Franciscan religious order), which encompasses the wisdom of a soul who understands the laws that govern the process of transformation:

> Lord, make me a channel of thy peace—
> That where there is hatred, I may bring love—
> That where there is wrong, I may bring the spirit
>   of forgiveness—
> That where there is discord, I may bring harmony—
> That where there is error, I may bring truth—
> That where there is doubt, I may bring faith—
> That were there is despair, I may bring hope—
> That where there are shadows, I may bring light—
> That where there is sadness, I may bring joy.

Through transformation, we receive the enlightment that allows us to know ourselves on a deeper level. We can glimpse the parts of ourselves we dislike and judge as bad; we can also glimpse our essence and begin to remove the barriers to healing. This enlightenment grows as our awareness continues to expand. While some people benefit from professional psychotherapy, that *alone* rarely brings the fulfillment that comes from knowing one's own higher power. Expansion of awareness involves taking inventory, so to speak, of all that is inside us, including all the emotions, past traumas, resentments, painful memories, and guilt that exert their effect through our unconscious minds.

THE CONSCIOUS AND UNCONSCIOUS

To a great degree, we live our lives under the control of parts of ourselves that lie in the unconscious. Awareness is the ability to witness our lives and unconscious behavior in a nonjudgmental way without the immediate need to control things. For example, a woman is depressed after learning that she has breast cancer. She feels unattractive and unlovable at the thought of her body after a mastectomy. She shuts herself off from her husband and her children. She is raging inside about how life could do this to her. She is overcome by depression and rage. There is no awareness, no reaching toward a new perspective—only complete identification with her anger. However, once she can bring the depression and rage to her objective awareness, she can experience them, rather than just avoid them, and then observe these powerful emotions impartially.

Without this awareness, she identifies so strongly with her pain because she doesn't see she is more than these emotions, and she acts out her anger and fear in ways that are destructive and hurtful to herself and those closest to her. This unaware expression is called identification: by being unaware and unconscious of her emotions, she totally identifies with them, trying to avoid the pain associated with them. By pushing them deeper into the unconscious, she continues to allow their destructive power to be manifest.

Another way we remain unconscious of parts of ourselves we dislike or judge as bad is to disown them. This is our attempt to eradicate those aspects and traits we consciously dislike or have been taught are bad, driving them deeper into our unconscious. As mentioned in chapter 6, Carl Jung described these disowned parts or selves as "the shadow." For all of the selflessness, humility, courage, and morality we cultivate, we simultaneously create the shadow of jealousy, conceit, fear, and violence, driving into our unconscious a whole array of unwanted "selves."

Jung also wrote:

> To become conscious of [the shadow] involves recognizing the dark aspects of the personality as present and real. This act is the essential condition for any kind of self-knowledge and it, therefore as a rule, meets with considerable resistance. Indeed, self-knowledge as a psychotherapeutic measure frequently requires much painstaking work extending over a long period. Identification, then, is the expression of unconscious patterns with such force and emotion that we are not only unaware of this acting out but powerless to control it. At other times we drive disowned, unwanted parts of ourselves so deeply into our unconscious that they must manifest in destructive ways.

Sal: Negative Energies and Cancer

■ Sal developed testicular cancer at the age of twenty-eight. He had graduated from law school a year before his diagnosis. He strongly identified with the religious, spiritual side of himself, and he told me that he thought selflessness was the highest attribute and that his goal was to use his legal knowledge to bring justice to those who could not afford it. His concern was for the powerless in society, and he had originally entered law school with the intent to help the homeless through work in urban development and planning.

Sal's philosophy had always been that by learning to control his negative energy and by acting in a selfless, kind way, he would find fulfillment. After graduation, he worked for a firm that dealt with the city and state in public housing and real estate law. Soon after starting, he was shocked to see the dishonesty and greed around him. He worked on one case after another, each time disappointed that his clients and the other lawyers "were only out for themselves and the almighty dollar."

Having disowned his own power, dishonesty, and greed, Sal could not see these traits in his colleagues until it was too late.

I asked Sal to focus and meditate on the shadow of his selfless, generous self. That night, he had a dream.

"I was walking home from work and took a wrong turn down a dimly lit street," he told me. "From behind a car, a gladiator with fierce strength and ice-blue eyes jumped out at me with a sword. He stood in front of me. I turned to run the other way, and there he was again, facing me with his sword unsheathed and ready to strike at me. I woke up in a state of panic."

Sal's dream reveals the degree to which he had so totally repressed and disowned a powerful part of himself. This powerful self may be depicted in dreams as a masculine self or a warrior. It has been called in various forms of dream interpretation "warrior energy" or the "warrior archetype." Sal's warrior energy had been repressed since childhood and was now conveying to his consciousness that it was angry with him.

The warrior archetype and other instinctual energies and archetypes are within us all. They will not stay repressed permanently—they may come out in the form of illness or a variety of other ways. By becoming aware of these energies, we allow their expression on a conscious level, rather than confining them to an unconscious plane where they may manifest themselves in destructive ways. Like Sal, if we cannot see the dishonesty and greed in our own lives, we will not see it in others, and we will find ourselves in relationships with dishonest, greedy individuals, as Sal did. By remaining unaware of our shadow energies, we make ourselves vulnerable to those people who reflect the energies we have disowned.

In one of our meetings, Sal recalled how, when he was a young child, his mother had enrolled him in parochial school the day after he had been involved in a fight with another child in his public school. She had told him, "You must not fight, no matter who is right or who is wrong."

While a mother's protectiveness is understandable, not allowing Sal to deal with his instinctual aggression resulted in years of repression of his masculine warrior energy. Sal's parents also consistenly prohibited him from enrolling in contact sports like football, which he loved to play and watch. I do not believe it is a mere coincidence that he developed cancer of a male sexual organ.

Sal completed his radiation therapy successfully, and he also began to embrace his instinctual power. He left his law firm and became a successful litigation attorney.

On a recent two-year routine checkup, he told me, "In law school, I would never have considered being a trial attorney, because the whole concept gripped me with fear and revulsion. At the time, I thought it was beneath me, and not consistent with my spirituality and higher morality. I looked down on my fellow students who wanted to do this, out of my own fear of power, which I could not even face. I've come to realize more fully that I haven't had to compromise my ideals or principles in the process of embracing my entire being. I can see the world and myself for what they are—the good and the evil, the greedy and the giving, the conceited and the humble. Once I could stop judging and just start observing this first in myself and then in the world, nothing seemed so bad, nothing seemed so fearful."

FORGIVING, NOT DISOWNING

Disowning parts of ourselves can not only result in physical illness and fear but also prevent us from expressing the yearnings and passions in our hearts. Becoming aware of our unconscious "selves" and motives, we begin to understand the origin of many of our destructive emotions, such as depression, fear, and frustration. Until we can see our unconscious destructive patterns, they will continue to cause suffering and distress in our lives, and keep us from discovering the peace, love, and serenity of our essence. As we become aware of our essence, we can discard our feelings of emptiness and insecurity, as well as much of our fear. Our fear of loss can result in greed. Our fear of being vulnerable can result in needing to feel superior to others. Our fear of being unlovable or of being rejected can result in an obsessive drive toward perfection and success.

When we discover our essence, love replaces fear. When we let go of fear, we begin to glimpse our higher self. This process of discovery requires two major attributes: honesty and humility. We must be willing to examine our lives with detachment and honesty. To do this, we must have the humility to accept that we are not perfect, that we have harmed others, and that we have plenty of room to grow.

Humility comes when we let go of conceit. We have conceit because we have fear. Many of our deepest fears, such as those of rejection and worthlessness, begin when we are children. We react to these fears, even though we may be unconscious of them, in part by becoming conceited.

Conceit can take many forms: we may feel superior to others, we may seek power over others, we may even manifest violence against others in "accepted" ways, such as through competition. I am not referring to the competition of a sporting event, but to economic or business competition in which we leave our competitors ruined and demoralized. People in contact with their essence who have found humility never act this way.

We also need to find the love and forgiveness in our hearts. Forgiveness provides us the context for deeper realizations, which come when we understand that we were never supposed to be perfect. We must allow ourselves to forgive our wrong actions, imperfections, illness, and those who have wronged us. Forgiveness is a state of mind that sees through the eyes of the soul all that seems imperfect in the world and in ourselves. Thus, what is imperfect can provide us with lessons we need to learn and direct us to find the source of true compassion. Forgiveness leads to healing insight, which allows us to learn from our mistakes and still be compassionate with ourselves.

Disowning parts of ourselves can lead to destructive behavior, depression, lack of fulfillment, and physical illness. Only by expanding our awareness to encompass our entire being in a spirit free from judgment and resistance can we remove any barriers to the love and joy of our essence. Transformation allows us to be aware of opposite forces within us and to heal the tension that exists between them. The physician-healer should be able to assist the patient in beginning to find and surrender to his or her essence, so that healing can begin.

Patients must also learn to accept healing at the level of their essence, so that the drugs, radiation, or any other medical therapy may work as well as possible. I have seen many patients who, on a conscious level, wanted to recover their health, while on an unconscious level were on an opposite path. These patients saw chemotherapy and radiation therapy as darkness rather than light, and they developed much more severe side effects than those patients who saw the positive, healing powers of their treatment.

John: Unconscious Darkness and Hodgkin's Disease

∎ John had noticed a swollen gland in his neck. A biopsy confirmed an initial diagnosis of Hodgkin's disease, which is curable with radiation and chemotherapy in about 90 percent of patients when it is caught in the early stages.

"I think all your chemotherapy and radiation is just poison that destroys the immune system," he said.

John, a psychologist, was quite knowledgeable about his disease. Over the previous two years, he had seen five oncologists before me, in addition to doctors practicing other alternative forms of therapy. He had tried several nontraditional forms of therapy, including herbal therapy, high doses of vitamins, and macrobiotic diets. They all had failed, and his disease had progressed.

"I guess I don't have any choice but to take a chance on your poisons killing me," he said.

Although very reserved about his family life, John told me he had a strained relationship with his father, who was controlling and always "meddling in *my* decisions about my life." I tried to explain to him, especially since he was a psychologist, the need for honesty and self-examination as a starting point. I pointed out to him that his disease, having progressed from an early to an advanced stage, was his major problem, not modern medicine: the major risk to his life was his disease, not my "poisons." I asked him to examine his anger at doctors, his illness, and his father. He should try to see how his view that medicines were poisons could likely be self-fulfilling. I also suggested he see a psychiatrist for help in dealing with all these issues.

"For one, I'm a psychologist, and a psychiatrist can't tell me anything I don't already know," John answered. "And two, I'm going to go see another doctor who will just get this over and done with."

Patients with more severe side effects from chemotherapy and radiation often have deep-seated unconscious anger and resentment of parental figures such as doctors. This anger and resentment frequently result in a host of destructive feelings and thoughts, accumulated over a lifetime, being projected onto the doctor, as well as the therapy. The sudden expression of these repressed energies can result in more severe vomiting, hair loss, and other side effects during cancer treatment.

Subsequently, John developed every major side effect to both the chemotherapy and the radiation. He refused bone marrow transplantation, which was recommended by his new doctor, and he died of his disease.

You may ask how "poisons" such as chemotherapy or radiation can have any relationship to your essence or healing. Martin Buber asked the same question in a parable in *Tales of the Hasidim*: "But why does one give poisons to the sick?" And he answered:

> The "sparks" that fell from the primeval inquity of the worlds into the "shells" and penetrated the stuff of stones, plants, and animals—all ascend back to their source through the sanctification of the devout who work with them, use them, and consume them in holiness. But how shall those sparks that fell into bitter poisons and poisonous herbs be redeemed?

That they might not remain in exile, God appointed them for the sick: to each the carriers of the sparks which belong to the root of his soul. Thus the sick are themselves physicians who heal the poisons.

Matter and spirit are energy, and they are intimately linked. On a conscious level, John wanted to be cured of his disease, but on an unconscious level he was unable to see how his preconceived ideas and anger prevented him from seeking appropriate therapy. Also, he was not willing to acknowledge or rely on his essence to guide him in his quest to find healing.

Jung wrote:

It is often tragic to see how blatantly a man bungles his own life and the lives of others yet remains totally incapable of seeing how much the whole tragedy originates in himself, and how he continually feeds it and keeps it going. Not consciously, of course—for consciously he is engaged in bewailing and cursing a faithless world that recedes further and further into the distance. Rather, it is an unconscious factor which spins the illusions that veil his world. And what is being spun is a cocoon, which in the end will completely envelop him.

THE DOCTOR: RAISING CONSCIOUSNESS

I always try to release patients from their preconceived ideas and fears about chemotherapy and radiation therapy by first helping them become conscious that their fear exists. This basic fear tends to drop by the wayside when they see the therapy as an ally and as light. Some patients even wish to take their medication in their hands and acknowledge it as an absolutely positive substance before taking it into their bodies. Most of these patients experience far fewer side effects and even tend to respond more positively to the therapy.

By failing to recognize the existence of the unconscious aspects of patients, doctors deny the importance of those aspects. Yet physicians could help their patients become more aware of the complexities that the unconscious mind contributes to an illness and to the healing process. And once physicians see and understand the importance of this dynamic in the healing process, it will become part of the traditional healing process. That recognition also would lead to changes in the way doctors run their busy practices. Doctors must realize that their current healing tools are of limited value if the patient's unconscious makeup is ignored or the patient's need to be aware of his or her essence and purpose is ignored. The physician's goal must be to allow patients to receive healing on physical, psychological, and spiritual planes. This is done by allowing patients to see that aspects of both their mind and their essence may be using illness to resolve certain conflicts and learn certain lessons. Patients must then be allowed to see the very real possibility of resolving these conflicts and learning these lessons by embracing healing rather than retreating from the lessons.

CONSCIOUSNESS THROUGH ESSENCE

Your conscious mind identifies with your thoughts, emotions, and body to the point that you feel, "I am my thoughts. I am my sadness and fear. I am my body and illness." When you can see and then release these conditioned thought patterns and begin to experience the fact that you are more than your thoughts, emotions, and body, you begin to let go of all that is blocking healing. When you can remove the wall you have built around your essence, what is left is your essence. When you can see and then let go of the illusions you have been so identified with, all that is left is your truth. When you can surrender your attachment to fear and suffering, all that remains is healing. You have been so afraid to let go of all these things, because you fear there will be nothing remaining to hold on to. Surrender requires the trust to just let be. Confucius said, "You cannot create a statue by smashing the marble with a hammer, and you cannot by force of arms release the spirit or the soul of man."

You know that wisdom is seeing the world through the eyes of the soul, which you come to know through ESSENCE healing. When you identify with your essence, you may see adversity and illness as necessary teachers rather than as unexplainable curses. Perspective allows you to see how many others have suffered far more than you. You may know this is true and still surrender to the fact that you were never meant to know why. In this context, healing is not so much concerned with fighting and struggling against illness. Rather, it begins by surrendering illness—and your reactions to it—to your essence. Healing then becomes a fight that you cannot lose.

Your essence has a wonderful melody, and its light imparts an energy you may not have experienced previously. Feeling the power within your essence gives you a sense of freedom from your problems and suffering. No matter how deep the depression, how serious the illness, how hopeless the problem, you can discover a new meaning and experience a new reality in your life. Such a discovery can and does occur in brief glimpses—this is why patience is required. But as a physician, as a healer, and as a soul on this planet, I have found no greater sense of wonder and satisfaction than by observing this transformation in people. No endeavor can bring a physician more fulfillment than assisting people in this healing process.

ESSENCE
Meditation:
Removing the Barriers
to Healing

■

This seven-step ESSENCE healing meditation allows people to begin removing their barriers to healing. The negative judgments you have about your illness create resistance, which is one of the greatest barriers to healing. We can think of it as a warm-up or practice guided meditation. Starting out, many of us find we have emotional barriers to looking inward. We need to remove these barriers so we can progress on our journey. This guided imagery meditation is designed to help us do that. The more we meditate, the more skill we develop at it, and the more adept we become at removing emotional barriers.

Begin by sitting on a couch or chair in a quiet place. Take several deep breaths. Slowly inhale deeply into your abdomen. Now slowly exhale as completely as you can. Concentrate on each breath. Breathe in through your nose and out through your mouth. With each breath repeat to yourself several of the following positive thoughts with the word *infinite* before them. For example, think of infinite healing, infinite truth, infinite light, and infinite peace. Visualize each breath being directed to a clear blue mountain lake located in the upper part of your abdomen or solar plexus. Then take two to three minutes to observe each breath without trying to control it.

1. EXPERIENCE

Experience how deeply troubled you are about an unwanted occurrence, emotion, or illness, and become aware of your anger and
resentment toward it.

Become more aware and realize how much you care about this
unwanted part of your life. Become conscious of your resistance
to it. If you deny that you care deeply about an unwanted occurrence, emotion, or illness, you deny yourself healing of a part of
you that may need it most.

If deep inside, you are ashamed, sad, or scared, this must be
healed before any other healing can occur. Think of this part of
yourself as a frightened child who requires care, not neglect. You
must experience the feelings about unwanted occurrences or illness
in your life, so that you can begin to heal them.

Say to yourself, "I wish to experience the hurt and sadness about
this occurrence. I have created this hurt and sadness by forgetting
my essence."

Spend a few minutes being open to any feelings and questions
that come forth. You might ask, "Where did the hurt and sadness
I'm now aware of come from? How have I forgotten my essence?"

2. SEE

See and realize how you are powerless to change the past or the
fact that the unwanted occurrence or illness has occurred.

You do not want to admit that you are powerless in any circumstance. You have learned that you need to be successful,
wealthy, healthy, and happy—anything but powerless. You have
pride in your abilities, your achievements, and your power to overcome adversity. Therefore, it is difficult for you to accept that life
occasionally provides you with realities you are powerless to stop.
You cannot simply wish away illness or the loss of a loved one.
You cannot rid yourself of it with alcohol or other avoidance mechanisms. However, you can come to understand your emotions associated with an unwanted reality. In turn, you can ask your

essence to transform your destructive emotions and reactions through wisdom.

Say to yourself, "I may be powerless to change the past, but I am no longer powerless to change my attitudes, thoughts, and outlook. I am no longer powerless to bring healing from my essence."

Contemplate this for several minutes and allow any questions and realizations to come forth. You might ask, "How does my realization that I am powerless to change this occurrence make me feel? If I have the power to bring healing from my essence, am I ever really powerless?"

3. SURRENDER

Surrender to the fact that the unwanted occurrence or illness is a reality and has occurred. While this point may initially seem obvious to you, it probably requires the most contemplation on your part to really accept and understand. Your conscious mind thinks, "Of course, I must accept it if it's already a reality."

The fact is, you do not accept unwanted realities so readily. Instead, your mind resists ("How could I be victimized by such bad luck?"), makes destructive explanations ("I've always been a failure, so now here comes just a greater one to top it off"), and becomes mired in sorrow and self-pity ("My life may as well be over—it's not worth going on just to have more of this").

Your mind rejects the *acceptance of* unwanted occurrences or illnesses and goes automatically to its old, negative, conditioned patterns. It is only by quietly accepting the unwanted realities in life that you can begin to grow and approach your essence.

Say to yourself, "I surrender to the fact that unwanted occurrences have happened in my life. I also surrender to the power of my essence to heal my reactions, thoughts, and attitudes about these circumstances." Spend a few minutes feeling the power associated with this thought.

Be aware of any realizations or questions that come up. You

might ask, "What is the difference between surrender and true power? What is true power?"

4. EMPOWER

Empower yourself to heal by bringing to your awareness and to your essence all emotions regarding and leading up to the unwanted occurrence or illness. Bring to your essence the guilt, anger, and fear, as well as any feelings of unworthiness, which may have contributed to the unwanted occurrence or illness.

Say to yourself, "I empower myself to remove the barriers I have created to healing. These barriers block me from knowing the vast power that lies within me." Contemplate this statement for several minutes and be aware of any questions that come up. You might ask, "How does my conceit keep me from seeing my true power? How may humility allow me to express my higher power?"

5. NURTURE

Nurture the realization and experience of the power within your essence. Become aware that there is a higher self or power within you that in some way not only can serve but can be served by the unwanted occurrence or illness. Contemplate that this higher power has the capacity to bring healing to the situation.

When confronted with an unwanted event or illness, you may feel that God is punishing you for something, or you may conclude that because of the unwanted event there must be no God. You may feel guilt that somehow the illness is your fault. However, awareness of your essence allows for these unwanted occurrences to be accepted with hope, trust, and understanding. You have an inherent reality that is your essence, and this essence may bring you to a closer relationship with whatever you conceive to be God. It can bring you wisdom and knowledge of universal truths. It can always experience healing.

Once adversity is accepted, you can begin to see the many ways you can transform. Perhaps an adverse occurrence reveals to you that you need to obey your heart more than your mind. Perhaps you need to spend less time working and worrying, and more time in solitude developing a new link to spirit. There are countless other paths for transformation that may be revealed to you. All adversity offers us a blessing in some form, no matter how ugly its disguise. This is also stated in the New Testament of the Bible: "And we know that all things work together for good to them that love God" (Romans 8:28).

Say to yourself, "I will nurture and cultivate my realization that my true power lies within my essence. I will look here for truth and purpose. I will look here for healing." Contemplate this statement for a few minutes.

Notice any realizations or questions that come forth. You might ask, "How can I nurture this reality so healing can continue? What will sustain and actualize this reality for me?"

6. CREATE

Create a space where you can embrace your soul in trust, so that all necessary lessons can be learned and healing can be given. This process is done in the solitude of your own heart through quiet contemplation.

Even though your mind resists the concepts of powerlessness and surrender, this is only because these concepts are often misunderstood. When you are powerless, you have the opportunity to surrender, and what you surrender to is your own essential power. You first let go of your mind's struggle. You can touch the power and energy of your essence through a quiet mind and an open heart. A quiet mind comes about by examining the origin of each thought. It is only by asking, "Is my thought about this occurrence based on my essence, or is it just another negative, conditioned thought pattern?" An open heart is reached simply by the intent to touch the source of your compassion. Feel the lightness of letting go, and embrace the energy of the soul. Surrender allows you to live in harmony with life, rather than wage an ongoing war against it. It is from this space that healing can come forth.

Say to yourself, "I will continue to create a space where surrender and transformation can continue. I will spend time in this space daily, for here I am totally safe." Spend a few minutes contemplating this statement.

Notice any questions that come to you. You might ask, "How do I create and protect this space? What other space has ever provided me with the safety for transformation to occur?"

7. EMBODY

Embody and actualize transformation of your mind and body by deeply feeling your desire for this to occur.

Say to yourself, "I will continue on the path of transformation. I will do this by living my life with an awareness of who I am. I will endeavor to learn my purpose each day."

Ponder this statement and be aware of any questions that come up. You might ask, "How does my essence see the meaning of this unwanted occurrence? What is my purpose right now?"

You may now wish to record any realizations or questions in a journal. You may proceed to the ESSENCE Guided Imagery meditation, or take a break and do this at a later time.

REMOVING THE BARRIERS TO HEALING: THE SEVEN STEPS WITH YOUR EYES CLOSED

Begin with the breathing exercise.

1. EXPERIENCE

Experience where in your body you feel the judgments, anger, or resentments you have about your illness. Feel their exact location, size, shape, color, and temperature. Visualize them as energy. Pick only one area of your body at a time.

2. SEE

Visualize the light of your essence located above the top of your head.

3. SURRENDER

Surrender your judgments to the higher power of your essence by visualizing their energy being released upwards into the light of your essence.

4. EMPOWER

Empower and strengthen this healing by recalling your essence. Again visualize the light of your essence flowing into the area you are working on.

5. NURTURE

Nurture the idea of a life free from negative judgments.

6. CREATE

Create a space for your higher power to continue to guide you by visualizing a channel through which the light of your essence can continue to flow in and the negativity you are working with can flow out.

7. EMBODY

Embody and externalize this healing by visualizing the light of your essence flowing into each cell of your body.

Part Three

THE FOUR PATHS OF HEALING MEDITATION

Path I:
Releasing Fear

Fear of the unknown is forgetfulness.
There is no such thing as the "unknown"
to the soul. There is a natural fear
and resistance when one does not recall
one's own Divinity.
   —*Pat Rodegast and Judith Stanton,*
   Emmanuel's Book

We are all born with two strong fears—a fear of falling and a fear of darkness. Both of these are instinctual fears, buried deep in the psyche. The fears I want to talk about are the dreaded but inevitable occurrences that most of us have been conditioned since birth to view as bad and to avoid. These are our fears of death, illness, rejection, and failure. Because of these fears, we think that illness cannot possibly have any benefit in our lives and that it certainly has no place in our spiritual existence.

But perhaps illness does have something to offer us. Fear of it may be a barrier keeping us from something positive. Further, fear itself can make us ill, so overcoming fear can be a step toward healing.

Letting go of fear is the first step in knowing the truth of your essence. Overcoming fear is not so hard once you understand it. We all think we know what fear is. When we face a distressing day at work, our heart rate may increase, our palms may sweat, and we may feel tightness in the stomach. Some people may even have panic attacks. When we have an illness, we may also feel anger. We may blame ourselves for not having done something to prevent it. We may feel as if we have nowhere to turn. The reactions that accompany these thoughts could be called fear, but none of these truly are fear—they are only the *illusions* of fear. They are the emotions that grip us when we avoid or try to escape from what we think we fear.

Ron: A Healing Soul and Lymphatic Cancer

▮ Ron was born with cerebral palsy. This condition left him with a hip deformity that required him to walk with the aid of braces and crutches. Despite his disability, Ron married, adopted two children, put himself through college, and taught handicapped children. Then at the age of forty-four, he developed lymphoma, a cancer of the lymphatic system. He first noticed this as a lump in his groin that caused massive swelling in his leg.

Having lived with the effects of cerebral palsy from such a young age, Ron had already developed a deep connection with his soul and the healing this brings. He told me, however, that doubt was beginning to creep into his mind. "I'm starting to wonder just how much one person can go through in a lifetime," he said.

I had Ron do several ESSENCE Guided Imagery meditations over the following week. He told me at his next visit, "I realized as a child there were no guarantees that my life was ever going to be a certain way. I understood this completely free of fear. Only after having to face this new challenge of cancer, however, did I see *why* there need be no fear. During a meditation yesterday, I experienced strongly the feeling that there was no guarantee for safety in this world. I also experienced the fear I now had about this. Then I simply surrendered to this sense of reality. I did not surrender to the fear; I surrendered to the reality. This feeling of surrender immediately allowed me to get back in touch with who I am, and feel the inherent safety within my heart."

Ron was determined to overcome this illness. He began treatment with chemotherapy. His pain and struggle just to go for tests and treatments were more than many other people could have borne. However, my other patients saw Ron come into the office each time with a cheerful attitude. They began to realize how much power they had to react more positively to their own illnesses, too. After talking with Ron in the waiting room, one of my patients who was receiving chemotherapy for breast cancer told me, "I feel ashamed of myself for my self-pity and anger. Here was this man listening to *my* story with such complete attention and then offering *me* words of encouragement."

Ron used his own pain to heal those around him. Several people I have known have had an impact on the lives of others out of what they learned through their own pain. I asked Ron if he realized the degree to which he influenced those around him. He answered, "I have no question about how much my life means or what it is I am here to do."

Ron went on to have a rapid, complete remission of his lymphoma, which has now lasted over two years. He is, in all likelihood, cured. As the deaf and blind educator Helen Keller wrote, "To keep our faces toward change and behave like free spirits in the presence of fate is strength undefeatable." Souls such as Ron's can truly heal.

HIGHER POWER

We like to think our greatest fears lie in those things over which we have no control. They do not. The things we really fear are looking directly at the wall that surrounds our own essential power and looking at the power itself. We fear both so much that we are not even conscious of their existence. This power is not the kind of power we are accustomed to thinking about, which involves controlling things or dominating others. I'm referring to our higher power, which emanates from our essence.

For a person to glimpse such power, it is necessary to know the soul. The soul is where *true* power emanates from. To see the world through the eyes of the soul is to know that in all this world there is nothing to fear.

The civil rights leader Martin Luther King, Jr., embraced this power. Although he was aware of the danger he faced in the quest for equality and human rights for all, he transcended his fear. He could have been content to teach only the parishioners of his local church, and would then have likely lived out a long, comfortable life with his family. But where most of us would have let our fear keep us from embracing such power, he understood that it could transform a nation. In his short life he changed the world. But power and vision are not reserved for those few who achieve greatness. Such greatness is in us all. We just need to remember it is there.

Thus, we should reexamine the need for safety from a different perspective. The concept we have now about safety is one in which we have only the "good things" in our lives while we keep out the "bad" ones. However, being open to our essence requires that we be open to all of life. It requires we also be open to the suffering in the world. It is not possible to experience only the inner peace that comes with opening your essence while being closed to the world. Both can be experienced together. In Taoist philosophy it is taught that to know heaven, we must also know earth; to know light, we must also know darkness; to see the positive, we must also see the negative. Thus, openness can replace safety, just as fearlessness can replace courage. When we operate from our essence, we experience a sense of surrender that allows life to unfold through openness and fearlessness.

Once our mind looks inside the wall surrounding our essence, we can see and feel the higher power that rests within. Then we can do all of the things we've wanted to do but were afraid to. We would no longer be afraid to ask, "Is this what life is really about? Is struggle all we are here for—just to make a living? Have we been living our lives totally unaware of a deeper purpose and meaning?" By asking these questions and looking inside that wall, you will be able to see the truth behind all the things you have feared, and will feel free to embrace what you've been avoiding. In so doing, you will release your fear—your fear will die.

No part of you consciously wants to die, however, and your fear is no different. But this fear is an entity you have created and empowered during every waking hour. This is not your instinctual fear, but the fear you've been taught since childhood. You give so much power and devote so much energy to it, that it has taken on a life of its own. And in allowing it to take over your life, you've created a life based in fear. The wealth, success, and comfort you think you have are actually based in the fear of losing them. You also worry about many things that will never even happen. What happens when you figure out that what you were worrying about will not happen? You start worrying about something else that probably will never happen. As the novelist A. J. Cronin wrote, "Worry never robs tomorrow of its sorrow; it only saps today of its strength."

FEAR AND POWER

We fear things our forebears simply and wisely accepted as part of life. What we mean by "comfortable" is the avoidance of any pain, difficult challenges, or events that "try one's soul." We have created the illusion that life can and should be lived on a level that is impossible to achieve. But we will experience loss; we will sometimes fail; we will die. The English poet John Keats described the value of the trials we inevitably must face in life in the poem "Endymion":

> But this is human life: the war, the deeds,
> The disappointment, the anxiety,
> Imagination's struggles, far and nigh,
> All human; bearing in themselves this good,
> That they are still the air, the subtle food,
> To make us feel existence.

Life's trials and occasional worries do "make us feel existence," for they are as much a part of life as the comfort we have been taught to seek. What we have forgotten is that we have a powerful soul that can give us wisdom and healing during difficult times.

When we glimpse our soul, we are empowered.

One of my patients described this empowerment: "[It was] a feeling like I'd never known. I felt, for the first time, I could surrender to my oneness with God and the world." In *The Mark*, Maurice Nicoll wrote, "And if life were sweet and beautiful, without pain or misery, there would be no incitement toward self-creation, no struggle whereby we come to recognize the finer ingredients we possess and separate them from the coarser." When we are empowered enough to embrace the world and all of our being, we have clarity. Clarity allows us to see ourselves and our world free from fear. Once we have this clarity, we will never be afraid again.

Power that arises from the soul allows for the creation of new attitudes and new realities. Fear not only blinds us from seeing our own power but also keeps us from being open to the possibility of new attitudes that can empower us. As we begin the process of surrender, we embrace with trust all that is going on in our lives, good and bad. We embrace our fear, and perhaps for the first time truly experience it. This surrender is a process done quietly in our own heart, and it is one of the key points to learn in healing.

Do you find this concept difficult to accept? Don't deny any resistance you have to it. Our fear uses all the self-deception, trickery, and enormous energy at its disposal to keep us from seeing our own power. Part of the problem is that we want our fear. But in wanting it, we must also expect the inevitable discomfort it brings.

We don't know our own power because we've spent our whole lives giving it up and diminishing it. We give our power to others: to our bosses, spouses, and doctors. Parents and teachers, unaware of *their* own power, taught us that we had none. Society attempts to take our power by teaching us that conformity brings rewards and nonconformity is its own punishment. Advertisements sell us on what a perfect body should look like, how important it is to own a car, and how glamorous smoking is. We've come to believe that decisions about our lives are made by others.

Nonsense. We control what we eat, what we teach our children, how much violence we will go to see at movies, and what destructive explanations we will use to make sense of the world. If we feel we don't have joy, freedom, and love in our lives, we must ask why. We must find the source of the rules we live by. We need to ask why our lives are not as fulfilling as we feel they should be. We need to ask who gave us our values and expectations. We must honestly look back and ask how fulfilled our parents and teachers were who taught us the world was a certain way. How much joy, freedom, and love did they really experience? And can we give our own children more than this?

We have all disowned and forgotten various parts of ourselves, but mostly we have disowned and forgotten our power, and an awareness of our essence. What does this lack of awareness of our power and essence have to do with fear? Fear is forgetting; it is what we created when we forgot who we were. Discovering the truth within your essence is remembering. When we became detached and unaware of the essential power within our essence, we let others define who we were and what our lives were about. We learned that we were created in sin and that we were here to suffer, that we should fear God and the world, and that we were unsafe. But we learned that in possessions, success, and achievements we could find safety. However, we became only more disappointed and fearful when we found that our possessions, wealth, and achievements only engendered more fear. This is what the naturalist and philosopher Henry David Thoreau meant when he wrote, "The mass of men lead lives of quiet desperation." Most of us go through life unaware of our power, our potential, and the natural state of joy that we were meant to experience.

KNOWING AND LETTING GO OF FEAR

In order to let go of fear, we must first know fear. We must be afraid many times and live with our fear, but despite this, live with a determination to continue to learn and to love. To experience fear fully, we must stop avoiding it. We must allow ourselves to experience it without the need to avoid or escape from it. You will find that this experience is not only less frightening, but takes much less energy than the experience of constantly avoiding or escaping from fear. Helen Keller wrote, "Avoiding danger is no safer in the long run than outright exposure. Life is either a daring adventure or nothing."

The ESSENCE process is designed to assist you first in fully experiencing your fear and then in releasing it. Fear may cause you to shut down to life, turning living into just existing, so that you are separate from and unaware of your essence. Then you will then be afraid of life itself, and too afraid either to learn or to love. If fear stops you from either of these, you are beaten, for you will stop seeking the truth inside your soul, since that will have become too terrifying an endeavor.

There is more danger in this consequence of fear than in fear itself. If you become unable to embark on life's journey of trans-formation, then fear has overcome you. And such defeat is often permanent. This is why patience and courage are such essential virtues. Even if you still harbor a number of fears, you must not allow them to cause you to waiver. Continue to embrace life, even with all your fears. Never avoid situations or experiences that you know in your heart are necessary for your own healing and growth. Continue to learn the lessons necessary for your soul's evolution, despite your fears.

Once we allow ourselves to experience fear fully, we no longer lose energy in efforts to escape from it. Once there is no separation between us and our fears, we become our fear and do not need to do anything to avoid it, and fear ceases to be. Then we realize that we have never really known fear, only the avoidance of fear, and that we have come closer to knowing the truth of our souls. In short, we have achieved clarity.

CLARITY AND WISDOM

While fear is forgetting, remembering brings clarity. Clarity comes about through the realization that almost all the fear in our lives is an illusion—an illusion based on powerlessness. Powerlessness itself is an illusion, and one that we all must let go of at some time in our lives. As children, we all had numerous occasions when we felt, and were shown, how powerless we were. We were dependent on others for food, warmth, shelter, and love. We assumed we were powerless, and many of us still assume so, either consciously or unconsciously.

When we begin to experience the timelessness and security that lie within our essence, the illusion of powerlessness begins to fade. We start to see we have never truly been powerless for even a moment in our lives. Clarity is the result of allowing such illusions to fall by the wayside. With clarity, we see how our lives have been shaped by the decisions we have made, and we get an overview of all the things we have attracted through our essence. Fear then simply ceases. From this space within us, we can make the conscious choice to let go of fear.

Clarity can only be bestowed by your own essence. No one can give it or teach it to you. No one can ever take it away from you. When you have achieved clarity, you see all challenges and events clearly and without fear. When you have clarity, you will never be afraid again.

While clarity is a wonderful attribute, it is also a powerful weapon. It must be treated with great respect and used cautiously, for clarity connects us with our inherent power and, like all power, this can be used foolishly and without wisdom. Great harm has been done to fellow human beings and the planet by those who have achieved clarity but not the respect that allows for its reverent use. Those who pollute our oceans and destroy our rain forests for their own financial profit use their power and clarity without wisdom or reverence. This separation of clarity from one's essence is described in the New Testament of the Bible: "For what shall a man profit if he shall gain the whole world and lose his soul? Or what shall a man give in exchange for his soul?" (Matthew 16:26). Clarity alone cannot enable us to know the truth inside our soul. Clarity can only bring us toward the truth of our soul when combined with wisdom.

Wisdom is not the same as knowledge. True wisdom has nothing to do with facts or logic. Wisdom is a way of seeing. It cannot be pursued or taught to another, even by those who have achieved it. Wisdom is seeing the world through the eyes of your soul. People who are wise are those who have released their fear. They approach the world and use their clarity and higher power with reverence, because they come from and emanate the light of their essence.

With wisdom also comes healing. Wisdom and healing are available for all of us to receive, but we must know not only how to ask for them but also how to receive them. We will suffer with fear until we realize that within our essence lies our power. With patience and persistence, we gain wisdom, and we find we no longer need to pursue what our essence has had all along.

Linda: Cancer and Guilt

■ Linda was diagnosed six years ago with uterine cancer that had spread throughout the muscle of her uterus. She had undergone a hysterectomy and examination of her lymph nodes, as well as radiation therapy after the surgery. I saw her for the first time five years later, when the cancer had recurred in her lungs. I reviewed with her the diagnosis and recommended chemotherapy and nutritional support. I asked her if she had any idea why she developed the cancer. Her answer was startlingly frank.

"I know exactly why," she told me. "Seven years ago, I decided I must die."

I was not amazed to hear this. Such decisions are not uncommon. But I asked her to explain.

"I'm married, with three grown children," Linda went on. "Eight years ago, I was traveling on business and met a man who lives about fifty miles from where I live. He was also married. We started an affair and both fell in love. Neither of us told our spouse. About ten months before I became ill, I was lying in bed one night thinking about how I could end the affair without hurting either my lover or my husband. I decided the only way was to die."

After we discussed other possible solutions, I asked her if she felt she deserved to die.

"No, not exactly," she answered. "But I do feel terribly guilty about the mess I've made of my life and the people I may still hurt."

"Would you consider telling your husband?"

"I couldn't bear to hurt him in that way."

Over the next few weeks, with counseling and meditation, Linda came to understand that it had never been her intent to hurt either her husband or the man she had been having an affair with. This markedly lessened her guilt.

Several weeks later, Linda had a profound experience during a meditation.

"I saw a white light above me that just appeared in my mind's eye," she told me. "I felt my consciousness moving toward it and into it. I looked down at my body and my life from this light, and saw this innocent being who never intended to harm another soul. I realized then all the unconscious assumptions I had made. I had always thought about life and destiny as retribution and punishment for past sins. Now, I saw all the events in my life that I had attracted as necessary in order to teach me the lessons I needed to be in this light I was now experiencing. The current events in my life *were* based on my past—not in a vengeful way, but in a way that pointed out perfectly the illusions that had been keeping me out of the light. My fear of God also became transformed as I saw all of my sins as only mistakes I made by not being in this light and realizing my reality."

Linda had truly experienced her essence. She could no longer carry around guilt. It was transformed to forgiveness, once she was able to see the illusions that had caused the guilt to develop. She continued to respond very well to her medical and nutritional therapy.

Several weeks after her experience with the light, she told me, "It's so clear to me that I've lived most of my life assuming I was this awful person, and that if anyone found out, I'd be permanently shamed. I made many wrong, hurtful decisions based on this assumption. I've examined my whole life these last few weeks. I've seen all my mistakes as just mistakes—not intentional sins. Most of all, I've forgiven myself. I really do not feel I need this illness any longer to teach me this lesson. But in a funny sense, I know I'd never have learned it any other way."

As of this writing, Linda continues with her remission.

Dave: Embracing Vulnerability in the Face of Cancer

When we are immersed in depression, rage, or despair, we often forget what these experiences represent and where they come from. We forget that they originate in our own mind. In fact, they are nothing more than projections of our fears. We must step back and observe what it is that we are identifying ourselves with. Only then can we hope to gain insight into our problems.

Dave was a very successful, wealthy Wall Street executive when he was diagnosed at the age of fifty-five with stomach cancer. He was a hard-driving chain-smoker who consumed alcohol and food to excess and had already been treated for two stomach ulcers.

He had recently been involved in a protracted legal battle with another brokerage firm. "They thought they had me," he said, "but I turned things around and kicked them in the ass." His wife had left him during his legal difficulties. "She couldn't take the heat," he said. "She had to get out when things got a little tough."

Dave's anger and compulsive need to accumulate wealth were evident. His constant stress and self-destructive habits also indicated his need to shield himself from a core that he unconsciously feared was terribly vulnerable.

I asked him to tell me about his childhood.

"My father was an alcoholic with an unpredictable temper," he said. "Nothing I did was ever good enough, and I was pretty much scared to death of him. My brother was five years older than me, and out of his own fear, he took everything out on me. I felt like I had nowhere to turn sometimes between the two of those bastards."

Dave left home at eighteen, joined the air force, attended college for two years, and then decided he "wasn't going to make twenty thousand dollars a year like those other jokers." He became a stockbroker.

Even after he learned of his stomach cancer, Dave was not at all interested in spirituality or awakening. The cancer had spread to several lymph nodes in his abdomen, and these were surgically removed. He could not see any benefit in giving up his complete identification with his power side. I asked him if he could begin to think about the vulnerable aspects inside of him. His answer reflected his "top-gun" personality: "I've overcome every challenge I've ever been faced with, so how vulnerable can I be?"

Dave found out just how vulnerable he was six months later when a routine CAT scan showed that the cancer had spread to his liver. This was subsequently confirmed with a liver biopsy. Only then did he begin to experience the full force of what he had repressed for so long. He came into my office one day crying like a scared child and said, "I've failed. My wife is gone. My children don't speak to me. I haven't talked to my brother in twenty years. I don't even know anyone who isn't afraid of me who I can talk to, and now I'm going to die."

All this repressed energy took over at once. The challenge for me was to help Dave bring to his awareness both his power and his vulnerability. I encouraged him to begin to use the ESSENCE guided imagery process to meditate on his vulnera-

had just forgotten my soul. I never meant to be distant; I had just forgotten how to be close. I forgot that I'm not going to be here forever—that life is just a short visit. I'm sorry for the pain I've caused you and your mother."

Stan broke down in tears as he saw the father he had never known. He and Dave embraced. They talked the whole night about the past—and the future.

Dave fought the good fight in his battle with cancer. He responded well initially to the chemotherapy, and he was able to continue working for a year. He died eighteen months later.

At his funeral, Stan said, "Dad did the best he could for everyone here. We all know he was never perfect. None of us are. But I also know he always tried. He struggled with his pain and tried to show how he loved us the only way he knew how. I love you, Dad. I think your greatest gift to me was allowing me to tell you this before you died. Your love will live through me and all your family. You will live in all our hearts."

Martin Buber wrote in *Ten Rungs*, "Man is afraid of things that cannot harm him, and he knows it; and he craves things that cannot help him, and he knows it. But actually, it is something within man he is afraid of, and it is something within man that he craves." Dave realized that it was not the threatening world he was afraid of, but rather his attachment to fearful illusions that he alone had spent a lifetime creating. It was not money, position, and power he craved, but the experience of discovering the simple truths contained within the reality of his essence. The resolution of Dave's fears, as well as his lifelong quest for happiness, was found within himself—not in the outside world, where he had spent most of his life searching.

Pam: Self-Acceptance and Antibodies

■ We may not like change, but a change of direction away from fear and toward the soul always brings light and love. It allows us to come home to the truth inside our heart. This is, and always has been, our natural state. We may have been unaware of it, and our actions may have been far from this truth. As we find tolerance for competing opposite energies within our personality, life may actually become more complicated, but also more fulfilling and rewarding.

One's essence manifests its power. If we repress this, then the energy may be expressed in an aggressive way. We need to develop openness in acknowledging our soul's purpose and truth. For those who surrender to their essence as it makes itself known in their lives, life becomes a rich, uplifting, and joyful adventure. For those who resist it, their essence can only make itself known through fear, depression, or illness.

Pam, a twenty-year-old college student, was a competitive swimmer. She developed a disease called ITP, or idiopathic thrombocytopenic purpura, three years ago. This disease is characterized by antibodies being formed against blood platelets, which are important in allowing blood to clot normally. Most often the disease goes into remission with surgical removal of the spleen.

Pam's disease did not respond to surgery, and she required high does of steroids and other medications to control her disease. The medications' side effects were severely limiting her ability to swim competitively. She saw me for the first time two years into her disease, when she moved to New York City. I continued to adjust her many medications, counseled her, and introduced her to the ESSENCE guided imagery process. I asked her to try to focus the discipline, will, and power she put into swimming into the healing of her disease.

On her second visit, Pam asked me, "When will I be healthy enough to get back to full competition? Do you think I will be able to win the number of events I did before I became ill?"

Her drive and compulsion to win were evident from the anxiety with which she put her questions. I told her the answer to both questions could be found in discovering what it was inside her that caused her to be so driven to win.

Pam smiled and admitted she did not know. "I'll meditate on it and let you know next week," she said as she left.

The next week she told me, "I have been thinking about something that I haven't yet told you about because I rarely think about it in a negative way anymore. My brother, Rob, had an osteosarcoma [a cancerous bone tumor] of his left leg when he was seven. The leg had to be amputated. I was a year older than him, but we went to the same school. I was so embarrassed for myself, as well as for Rob, when I heard kids make fun of him behind his back. The jokes were so cruel. I had so much anger at a lot of the other kids and even at God for doing this to us." She began to cry. "But that is only part of the story," she said after a few moments. "I've also begun to remember this week how bad I was to Rob. I remember a time when the doctors thought the cancer had spread, and I imagined how my life would be better without him. I felt so guilty and evil for thinking this that I never told anyone."

Pam had lived a life of fear—fear that others would see the evil person she thought she was. She felt guilty about the shame she felt around other children. She felt guilty about some of the immature but human thoughts she had had as a child. Pam tried to hide her shame and guilt by denying the things she had been ashamed of. The awards, trophies, and accolades she craved never brought her the intended solace or fulfillment. Why? Because she always felt that they were intended for the person she appeared to be, not the person she really was.

Pam wrote the following in her journal after a meditation: "I have been living my life in fear. I fear failure because I fear rejection. I fear losing. When I'm sick, I can't compete—and I can't fail. I choose to heal all fear in my life."

Pam had actually come to know her essence from an early age. She had actualized her inner desire to swim and excel at athletics. But she also had encountered a common pitfall. While she had glimpsed her essence, she had assumed falsely that her essence was her entire self. Pam, like the rest of us, has a very human, imperfect self that has a lot to learn and plenty of room to grow. This human self has faults and shortcomings that we must accept in order to correct them. Even after we glimpse and come to experience our essence, with all its power and light, we still have our human side that requires healing and wisdom to grow.

Pam found she craved respect from others so much that she did not rest secure in herself. She found that the more she was able to respect her human aspects, the less she needed the respect of coaches, teammates, and classmates. She discovered that when she felt insecure, this affected not only her ability to compete but also her physical health. Her healing was based on the revelation that her own feelings of insecurity kept her from taking the constructive actions needed to work on herself.

"I now know that I don't have to be perfect in order to love myself," she told me. "I just need the perspective to see myself, my past, and my human mistakes from the viewpoint of who I really am. My pride has forced me to deny and try to escape my humanness. I created a fake self to cover this up. I've spent so much energy keeping this mask up, fearing people would see the person I really was—the person I rejected so long ago. Now I love my human self as well, and I no longer have to hide it. My need to win will no longer be based on the need to convince others I am better than I really am."

Three months later she was completely weaned off all medication. She remains in remission today and still swims competitively.

While the surgery and medication saved Pam's life, these alone were not enough. Having acknowledged the role fear played in every aspect of her life, Pam became aware of and released her fears. Completion of her healing could then occur.

ESSENCE healing allows you to discover and express the light within you. Listen to your essence—it is wiser than your intellect. Ask for guidance to bring you closer to and assist you in learning about the truth inside your essence, and receive whatever comes, free of judgment. As you touch your essence, you will also touch the divinity within you.

FEAR OF DEATH

I want to talk about one fear in more detail—our fear of death. We have been taught that life and death are opposites. This presumption allows fear to reign during the interval between birth and death. We are afraid of death simply because we don't know what it means to die, any more than we know what it means to live. We cannot know how to live until we know the truth of our essence.

Death is but another reality most of us would rather not think about. We know it is unavoidable, but we have not dealt with it consciously or surrendered to it in a way that can release the terror we have of it. We know death only through our fear of it, and we see it as something to be avoided. The word itself brings to mind not only fear but also symbols and ideas that have developed since childhood. Thus, we have a great deal to release before we can even think about death with a clear mind.

Letting go of our fear of death is a necessary step toward healing when we are confronted with an illness like cancer. Patients have transformed before my eyes from angry or fearful people to loving souls who see death, as one stated, as "another transition to be experienced." This is why healing fear is the first path of the ESSENCE meditation, for it brings the wisdom to see the world through the eyes of the soul. This healing is often associated with a deep realization that in all the universe there is not—nor has there ever been—anything to fear. When we come to realize this, we have to wonder why we didn't experience this awareness sooner.

When each of us was a fetus in our mother's womb, our needs were met. We existed in blissful, pure awareness. We had no desire to leave the womb and were free from fear. At birth, we were thrust from this warmth and silence into a cold, noisy, bright world. We were given no conscious choice about this, just as we are given no conscious choice about the time of our death. If death is a return, a rest, or whatever we conceive it to be, why fear it? Our essence is ready to give us the light of wisdom by asking. Our mind may be afraid of loss and the unknown, but our essence is secure. Our essence realizes that it came to this planet for a short visit.

The time of death in a person's life is important only to the mind. The mind cannot grasp eternity. It is fixated on whether one dies at a young or an older age. One's essence knows this is but another illusion of no real importance. However, I suggest that you not accept these attributes of your essence simply because they are written here. Allow your own realizations and truth to come into being as you do the ESSENCE meditations, for you must find your own truth.

It's not important for our mind to know whether there is life after death. It's not important for our essence to find out—it already knows. On a conscious level, it's really not important whether we believe one idea or another, because each belief has, as its shadow, doubt. Our doubt reflects our fear of the unknown. However, beliefs about life after death, the soul, or anything else may for some be a hindrance to truth. You don't have to believe truth for it to be true. Believing something to be true does not make it true. You do not have to believe what you read in this book—simply contemplate it in a way that allows the truth of your own essence to come through.

Death is the unknown. Fear of death is fear of the unknown. However, death need not remain unknown in this life. All we need to know of death can be revealed to us by our essence. While we have our thoughts and think we know who we are, such a perception is just another of our many thoughts. We also have thoughts about reincarnation and life after death, and we would like to know whether our thoughts about ourselves and our lives survive after death—will our worries, despairs, and desires survive our death? But we are far more than just our thoughts. Our essence exists on a level without thought, and we experience it through our heart.

From this experience, a new type of thought is created. We can begin to think with insight and perspective. This perspective allows us not only to see life with a truth that brings a new simplicity to it, but also to see which of our thoughts have deluded us into thinking they are so important that they can deprive us of peace, harmony, and freedom. Our thoughts of others' expectations of us, of separation, and of loneliness contribute to our view of the world as a fearful place. Our essence is ready to give us the insight to see that there is really no separation between life and death. We have created the illusion of separation, but it is just another thought that we can transform with insight. When we quiet our mind, our questions, fears, and beliefs about death are replaced as we touch our essence. This consciousness allows our mind to surrender completely to our essence with the deepest trust.

Our conditioning has never allowed us to ask whether our everyday struggle is actually *living* at all. We rarely ask whether living without joy, beauty, and trust every day is in alignment with how things should be, and in alignment with our essence. We have become accustomed to living life with anxiety and fear, and we look at death as just another thing from which to escape. But our essence knows that death and life are part of the same continuum. To live completely every day—as if it were a lifetime—can be done only by surrendering our attachment to those things that engender fear. Otherwise, we live a mechanical, conditioned existence and can never even ask what love and freedom are.

If we do not know how to live, we do not know how to die. Those who do not fear insecurity and loss see that life and death as separate ideas are only illusions, and that the endless circle of life and death is natural and beautiful. Realizing this, there is no need for security, and we know true freedom. When we live this way, no conflict exists, because we surrender our attachment to all that gives birth to fear in our lives; all our fears of the past die, and with them the expectations that cause us to fear the future. We can also die to the fears we have created through ambition and greed, and also to those fears we have avoided. The death of our fears brings a new innocence and joy, and gives birth to endless possibilities for our essence to live its truth.

To die, then, is to let our mind have freedom from attachment to the agonies and fears that constitute our daily struggle. This is why the breathing exercise I outline before each meditation is so important in allowing us to experience this circle of life and death. Symbolically, the *inspiration* (or in-breath) represents life, and the *expiration* (or out-breath) represents death. The moment between the two, if you can become aware of it for a fraction of a second, represents rebirth, transformation, and healing. Death, in this context, is the same as freedom. Thus, we need not fear death, but rather, allow our fear to die. Our fear of death lies in the need to avoid it, and rests, in illusion, like all other fears.

All negative, destructive feelings and thoughts are based in time. We are depressed about a past event or we worry about something that may happen in the future. Thoughts are, by definition, based in the past because they are rooted in memory. Although thinking is obviously necessary for us to function in society, the moment our thoughts lead to fear, depression, and worry, we rapidly drain ourselves of energy and, eventually, health. Our essence has a reality that is not the product of thought. Experiencing our essence leads to a new kind of thinking. We experience our essence—and simultaneously experience life without fear and without expectations. This leads to insight and perspective. The insight and perspective that come with ESSENCE healing can eventually transform all our thoughts.

ESSENCE
Meditation:
Releasing Fear

■

I developed this ESSENCE healing meditation to help patients become aware of their fears about illness, and heal them. The first path of healing fear is one of expanding your awareness of who you are and experiencing your inherent power. These realizations come about in the quiet of your own mind.

Find a quiet place to sit. It is best not to have music or other extraneous noise.

Sit comfortably on a couch or chair, with your eyes closed for two to three minutes.

Breathe deeply several times, inhaling into your abdomen as fully as you can, and then exhaling slowly all the air from your lungs. Breathe in through your nose and out through your mouth. With each breath repeat to yourself several of the following positive thoughts with the word *infinite* before them. For example, think of infinite healing, infinite truth, infinite light, and infinite peace. Visualize each breath being directed to a clear, blue mountain lake located in the upper part of your abdomen or solar plexus.

Spend another two or three minutes just observing your breathing without trying to control it.

First, work to heal the fear that bothers you most.

1. EXPERIENCE

Experience and feel that fear. Say to yourself, "I wish to experience my fear about . . . I wish to experience first the cause of my fear I see originating outside me."

You may feel the fear in your body like a pounding heart, or a tense feeling in your stomach.

Experience the fear in your body. Keep your attention in the areas in which you feel your fear.

What questions come up for you? You may ask, "How does my fear feel in my body? Does my fear originate within me or in a cause outside of me?"

If you find the fear you are working on too troubling, go to another that is less uncomfortable for you. You may need to work up to a particular fear with this healing meditation.

2. SEE

See the existence of a reality different from your current one. Behold the reality of your essence or higher power. Picture this reality as a light above you that is warm and pure, as something you wish to move toward.

Say to yourself, "I know there is an essence within me that has a different reality than the one I am currently experiencing." Allow questions to come to you as you ponder this statement. You might ask, "What might this reality feel like? How would awareness of this reality change my life?"

Allow yourself a few minutes to contemplate the statement and your questions. Remember, it is much more important to ask the questions than to answer them right now. Asking such questions with an intent to heal starts a powerful, creative, healing process within you.

Now say to yourself, "I intend to experience this reality of joy, love, and healing in place of my current one, which is based on illusion, fear, and negative emotions."

3. SURRENDER

Surrender to the power of your essence. Say to yourself, "I intend to surrender to the power that is in my essence." Allow any questions to come up as you contemplate this statement. You might ask, "What does surrender feel like? What does the power of my essence feel like?"

Create an atmosphere for this surrender to occur by thinking and feeling love and warmth. Imagine the peace and calm that rest within your essence, and say to yourself, "I am only in this physical body and this world for a short time. I surrender to that part of me that is eternal, loving, and at peace."

Allow any questions to come to you as you ponder this statement. You might ask, "Do I ever stop to think how short this life is? Is there more to this life than fear?"

4. EMPOWER

Empower your awareness to heal your fear. Shift your awareness to be in the light of your essence. Picture yourself looking from this light down onto your fears and fearful emotions.

Say to yourself, "My current reality will be here when I return, so for the next few minutes I allow myself to let go of and be free from my fear." Allow yourself to feel the separation from your fear and other negative emotions. Your intention here should be to step away from the emotional intensity of your fears.

Say to yourself, "With all the force of my will and intention, I direct this healing light to the fearful temporary illusion below that needs healing." What questions come up for you with this statement? You might ask, "Can my intention to heal really bring healing? Can my fearful reality be healed?"

5. NURTURE

Nurture and strengthen this intention. Say to yourself, "I direct the wisdom and energy emanating from my essence to clear the confusion and guide me to let go of fear and illusion in my life."

Allow yourself to ask any questions as you ponder this command. You might ask, "Where is there confusion in my life? What do I think I understand about fear that I really do not?" As you allow these questions to be asked, visualize the energy and light emanating from your essence. Direct it to your new reality, which is like a seedling that requires cultivation in order to grow.

Say to yourself, "I ask for this guidance to continue through my thoughts, dreams, the words of others, and events in my daily life."

Allow any questions regarding this statement to come forth. You might ask, "Have I received guidance from my unconscious before, when I was not expecting it? What guidance would be helpful to me now?"

You do not have to solve or cure anything. It is enough for you just to ask the right questions to initiate the creative healing process. There is no need to approve or reject what you are feeling.

Visualize again the bright light emanating down onto your fear and your illusory self.

6. CREATE

Create or conceive a new reality and way of seeing your life in place of your fear. Remind yourself that your fears are not real truth, regardless of the intensity of the emotions they produce. You must also remind yourself that you created your fear in the first place.

Say to yourself, "I have created my fear, and now I decide to let the light of my essence shine on this illusion."

You might then ask questions that arise, such as, "If I created fear with my thoughts, can fear disappear by changing my thoughts? If I am living from my essence, can fear still exist?"

7. EMBODY

Embody and incorporate your realizations into your current reality. Say to yourself, "When I am aware of my essence, fear cannot be a reality."

Allow yourself to ask questions that come up. You might ask, "Can I always be aware of my essence? What would my life be like without fear?" Further integrate this light into your reality by saying, "I have glimpsed the real truth that is my essence. In the face of this, my fear no longer has power over me. My ability and power to heal my fear are far greater than I ever suspected." These thoughts will further manifest a healing that will work long after the ESSENCE guided imagery process is complete.

Bring your awareness back to its original place. Know that it has been transformed by your light. Remember, healing happens bit by bit. Do not be discouraged if you are still conscious of your fear. You have overcome fear in your life before, even when you thought you could not. Your current fear is no different—it will dissolve as well.

As you heal certain fears, others may arise. Let them. As you learn the power of your essence to heal, you realize these fears can also be healed. Many of my patients work with compassionate psychiatrists, social workers, and psychologists. Do not deny yourself this type of professional help as well, if you or your doctor feel it may be beneficial.

You may now wish to record any realizations or questions in a journal. You may proceed now to the ESSENCE Guided Imagery meditation, or take a break and do this at a later time.

RELEASING FEAR: THE SEVEN STEPS WITH YOUR EYES CLOSED

Begin with the breathing exercise.

1. EXPERIENCE
Experience exactly where in your body you feel your fear. Feel its exact location, size, shape, color, and temperature. Visualize this as energy. Pick only one area of your body at a time.

2. SEE
Visualize the light of your essence located above the top of your head.

3. SURRENDER
Surrender your fear to the higher power of your essence by visualizing its energy being released upwards into the light of your essence.

4. EMPOWER
Empower and strengthen this healing by recalling your essence. Feel this as warm, healing light which you can direct with each in-breath, into the area you are working on.

5. NURTURE
Nurture the idea of a life free of fear.

6. CREATE
Create a space for your higher power to continue to guide you by visualizing a channel through which the light of your essence can continue to flow in and the negativity you are working with can flow out.

7. EMBODY
Embody and externalize this healing by visualizing the light of your essence flowing into each cell of your body.

Path II:
Going Beyond Suffering

Sweet are the uses of adversity,
Which, like the toad, ugly and venomous,
Wears yet a precious jewel in his head;
And this our life, exempt from public haunt,
Finds tongues in trees, books in the running brooks,
Sermons in stones, and good in everything.
—*William Shakespeare,*
AS YOU LIKE IT,
2.1.12–17

We all have to face suffering at some time. Confronted by illness, we react first by resisting it as an unwanted circumstance. This resistance may take many forms: we may try to deny our suffering, we may analyze it, or we may break down and cry. We may believe our suffering is a form of punishment for our failures, and we may angrily curse our fate. In any case, one of the most common reactions to illness is to judge it as bad, and this value judgment causes us to resist it. However, this resistance causes us more pain and more suffering.

GLIMPSING ESSENCE
THROUGH SUFFERING

I lost my own mother to breast cancer over thirty years ago, when I was nine years old. Several months after her death, I came to realize that as long as I failed to fully accept and surrender to the reality of her death, I would continue to suffer from her loss. I saw I was powerless to change the fact that she had been in great pain and died at a young age. I *could* continue to be angry. I *could* dwell on the fact that life was not fair—after all, the other children in my class had not lost *their* mothers. And I could have continued to dwell on wanting her back, along with life the way it had been. Instead, I glimpsed my own essence through this tragedy. I surrendered to the fact that I was powerless to change the past: she was gone. I surrendered to the power of my essence to heal the pain, and when I saw the peace and serenity this surrender brought, I felt empowered. I saw that while I could not control all the events I was faced with in life, I could choose how I responded and thought about them.

Unfortunately, many of us see how conditioned our own lives really are only when our illusions are disrupted. When we are successful at our career and have a happy family, with a loving spouse and children, we tend to be unaware of our conditioning. Only when there is a disruption in this illusion of security—such as illness, loss, or failure—do we realize the extent of illusion in our lives. Our need to avoid and resist any disruption in the illusion that we call our lives then becomes apparent. When we resist this disruption in our security, it invariably results in more pain, anxiety, illness, and depression. The problem with having and seeking better financial security, position in life, and possessions is that we are constantly afraid of losing them. Everything we acquire in the hope that we will have security has attached to it the shadow of fear. The more we have, the more we have to lose. And if we lose these precious things, we know we will suffer.

If we can see the danger of this conditioning, why don't we act to release it? The answer is that it is extremely difficult to negate what we have been taught and what we have assimilated since our childhood. To alter our thought patterns, our resultant behavior requires a courageous commitment to change.

The first step toward change that will alleviate our suffering is surrender. Surrender is the opposite of resistance. But it is a concept foreign to most of us, and the word itself has negative connotations. Rather, such phrases as "Don't give up," "Only the weak surrender," and "There is no such thing as 'I can't' " ring in our ears.

Such platitudes have been ingrained in us since childhood. The fact is that sometimes we *do* give up. Sometimes, in the face of overwhelming obstacles or pain, we really can't help but cry out. We cannot regain the power to lift ourselves up from adversity if we deny that it exists, or if we fail to experience it fully. What do we have to lose? What is the worst thing that could happen? Pain? Loss of money? Granted, these possibilities are very frightening, but what we fear the most is death. We expend so much energy in the form of fear over something as inevitable as tomorrow's sunrise.

SECURITY AND CONDITIONING

The only way to have the power and the freedom from fear that will allow us to respond to an illness is first to accept that the illness has happened, and to realize that we cannot change that fact. We must make a fundamental choice: either to be safe in our illusions, or safe in our essence. We cannot have both, for they are mutually exclusive. When we choose to be safe in our illusions, we choose safety in money, material possessions, ambition, and "all the good things in life."

To choose safety in these illusions is a choice based on fear. With that choice, we constantly seek that which we will eventually lose, and while we may have temporary happiness in the safety of such illusions, we still carry with us the shadow of fear. To choose safety in our essence is to realize that there is no safety in our illusions. Our essence needs no safety, and when we choose the safety of our higher self, all unwanted events in life are looked at from the viewpoint of our essence.

We can lose our possessions, our loved ones, or our jobs—this is part of the design of life. Yet we are told in advertisements, on television, and by other cultural means that there is security in money, achievements, and social status. Actually, security itself is an illusion, something unattainable. When we seek the impossible, we become upset, angry, and frustrated, for it is not the true nature of life or our essence to need or seek security. Insecurity is integral to life, just as change is: only that which is dead is secure. To be alive in this moment is to be insecure, as change is the very nature of life.

Our essence savors the unpredictable, but our mind holds onto the security of thoughts, desires, and worries, all based in either the past or the future. However, if we are to rejoice in life, then we must also rejoice in the insecurity of growth and change. Our pain lies in the need to cling to what we already know. Healing is like birth: it may be traumatic and shocking at first, but this is only because the mind holds onto its pain. Conversely, the more secure we try to become, the more dead we must feel. This is how we forget our essence. It is the nature of life—and of our essence—that we can choose to remember.

REJOICE IN UNCERTAINTY

The essence of living is in the unpredictable. In America, unlike most "less advanced" countries, we frown on any uncertainty in our lives. We like to prepare and make plans, reflecting our obsession with control, and our dependence only on what is known. In other words, society teaches us to stop the flow of life because of concern that we may not be able to control it. As individuals, we must examine how our own need for security causes us to be detached from the flow of life. We insure everything we can think of: our lives, bank accounts, houses, spouses, and cars. We insure ourselves on the emotional level, too. However, the more well insured we are, the more our very essence is suffocated in the process. Joy, meaning, and healing come from the new, the unpredictable, the person we happen to meet and fall in love with, or the child who comes into our lives and asks for nothing more than love. We must begin to realize that our fear of, and resistance to, change and unpredictability is a denial of the very nature and energy of life itself. We can stop resisting and start surrendering to this wonderful unpredictability by opening to our essence.

Since wisdom is seeing the world through the eyes of the soul, a person who approaches life with wisdom chooses safety in essence. When we discover our essence and its power, we have no need to seek illusory safety in greed, ambition, and possessions. Once we can simply observe life, realizing that unwanted occurrences are a necessary part of our existence and not inherently bad, we no longer need to resist it constantly. Then we can have the silence and peace necessary for the truth of our essence to be apparent. Experience of our essence allows basic faulty assumptions by which we have lived to drop away, and to heal the fear, the feeling of separateness, and the doubt that constitute suffering. Suffering leaves when we surrender to our essence, and it ceases when we can be vulnerable, trusting that our essence is totally safe and will guide our lives. Our essence allows us to begin to heal suffering by breaking the bond between unwanted events in our lives, and our illusions about why they occurred and what they mean.

I have found in treating patients with cancer that much of the pain they experience dissipates dramatically when they are able to let go of the resistance they have to their illness. This resistance to the reality of their situation can cause much more pain than the illness itself. We have discussed how most of us do not even know fear, sorrow, or loss—we know only the avoidance of them. If an illness only causes us to deny our feelings, then we will be neglecting a part of ourselves that needs healing. If we fail to first fully experience our feelings about an unwanted event or illness, affirmations that we can "beat it" will not allow us to evolve in a way that brings us closer to our essence. Positive thinking alone cannot bring inner peace and fulfillment. But discovering our essence can.

My Mother: Suffering and Surrender

I see suffering daily. Young fathers with advanced cancer come in for chemotherapy and, despite the pain, put on a smile for their family. They go home and to their jobs, trying to lead a normal life rather than focusing on their prognosis and their pain. I know the toll cancer takes on a patient and family from watching my own mother, who was diagnosed with breast cancer when I was seven years old. I remember her courage in taking the limited forms of radiation therapy available at that time. She knew what the outcome of her disease would be, but she had the faith and wisdom to accept it. This gave her the courage to spend as much time at home with her family as possible.

One day, I came home from school to find her screaming and gasping for air. I recall the helplessness I felt at the time. As the ambulance driver placed her on a stretcher for her last trip to the hospital, she told me, "Always remember that I'm not leaving you. I'll be with you each time you look up at the stars, in the sound of the wind in the trees, and in the quiet of the night as you sleep." These were the last words she spoke, and she died two days later in the hospital.

From my mother, I learned the lesson of surrender. As a nine-year-old, I saw how her suffering lessened as she accepted her illness and allowed her essence to continue to nourish and enrich me, my brother, my father, and herself. Over the next few years, I surrendered my own sadness to my essence, I saw how my own suffering was transformed to love and awe. I understood the beauty in the process of life and death, like the changing of seasons. In the words of the writer Katherine Mansfield, "Suffering can be overcome. . . . Everything in life that we really accept undergoes a change. So suffering must become love." Until we can learn acceptance and surrender, we continue to react unconsciously to events, and we react out of fear rather than out of love. Through surrender, we can learn to draw on our true power.

We think suffering is caused by an unwanted or tragic event, by our bad habits or gloomy view of the world. ESSENCE healing shows that our power lies in how we can transform ourselves. We may not be able to undo a tragic event, but we can evolve by changing our responses to it and thoughts about it, and allowing the light in our hearts to transform our attitude from despair to hope. We can let go of our resistance to a situation and accept it fully, and explore the space that seems foreign to us now. This is the space where we can surrender in total trust to our essence, and in this space, we experience freedom and joy.

Alice: Breast Cancer and Personal Worth

▌Alice was diagnosed as having breast cancer three years ago. At the time of her mastectomy, the cancer had spread to nine lymph nodes. Her sister had already died of breast cancer. Alice was terrified of the side effects of therapy. She was also afraid of dying. She became severely nauseated a full twenty-four hours before her therapy, a condition known as anticipatory nausea. This escalated and caused severe vomiting by the time she came into my office for chemotherapy. She completed the treatment, but her anticipatory nausea persisted, despite my attempts to allay her fear and counseling from a psychiatrist.

Six months after her therapy had been completed, Alice re-developed cancer throughout her spine and other bones. She again had severe nausea from her chemotherapy, and pain from the bone disease. Finally, she told me she was ready to try ES-SENCE Guided Imagery meditations. She had reached a point necessary for healing: she had an open mind and felt willing to examine painful thoughts and memories so they could be healed. Alice was "really ready" because she felt tangibly a deep desire for healing and she had the courage to let go temporarily of her conditioned ways of looking at herself and the world.

ESSENCE Guided Imagery meditations allowed Alice to

quiet her mind long enough to glimpse her essence and *experience* her fear, not just the struggle to avoid fear. She recalled how she had been verbally abused by her father repeatedly during fits of temper. "He used to scream at me for no reason," she said. "I even remember he woke me up when he came home drunk at 2:00 A.M. and accused me of sleeping with a boy in my class."

She experienced her sadness and her anger, and only then did she begin to glimpse her soul. She saw that her fear of her father had prevented her from committing to anything but short-term sexual relationships with men. She also saw that her wonderful childhood talent for drawing had been lost in the despair of her tormented home life. When she no longer had trouble meditating, she began focusing on her heart. She could see—without judgment—her anger, feelings of inadequacy, and conviction that she was unlovable.

Alice told me, "I assumed for so long that life was a certain way—the way I explained it to myself. When I glimpsed my essence, new and different explanations came to me. My father wasn't cruel, he just *acted* this way out of his own frustration. I was not ugly or bad—I just assumed this. The child in me assumed I must be repulsive for my father to have treated me the way he did. My fear of my father led to my fear of life. My fear of life kept me from being aware of who I am. It kept me from really living. But once I discovered my essence, I could no longer be afraid."

Alice began drawing and painting. She spent almost every evening watching sunsets and going for quiet walks in the park. One day she told me, with some embarrassment, that for a few minutes she felt the birds in the park were singing just for her. Finally she reached a point when she no longer required any medication for pain, and her nausea lessened dramatically. Now, she has lived with metastatic cancer in her bones for longer than most doctors would consider possible—three years—and she continues to live more fully each day than many of us do in a lifetime.

Alice felt humiliated because the love and affection she craved from her father was never bestowed. Instead, she was repeatedly rejected by him. She began to confuse the love and acceptance she desired with the person withholding it—her alcoholic father. As a child, she had begun to see her father as a desirable model because *what she craved from him* was worthwhile. She thus concluded that to be unlovable and distant—like her father—was a desirable goal. Although this may seem an illogical conclusion, to a child it makes sense.

After years of rejection by her father, Alice also concluded that to love is humiliating. So, as an adult, she felt that the most worthwhile way to live was to be free of emotion and to reject love. Since her father was the dominant parent, she also concluded that her loving mother was weak, while her withdrawn father was strong. (Most children, like Alice, tend to imitate on some level the "stronger" parent, and thus conclude that love, not other characteristics, is what makes a parent weak.) Alice thus withdrew from her essence and, gradually, her life. But once she discovered her essence and its emotional richness, she also began to see the attitudes and conclusions that had created her misconceptions. She saw how these misconceptions had caused her to live a life that betrayed the essence within her.

Was Alice suffering more *before* she opened up to her pain and personal tragedy, or *after* she could really experience them? The answer is, before. I can assure you, she has not suffered since—and Alice says that, too. The courage needed to seek our essence is tremendous, but it is available to us all if we know how to ask for it and how to receive it. The American philosopher Ralph Waldo Emerson expressed this lesson well:

There is a guidance for each of us and by lowly listening, we shall hear the right word. Certainly there is a right for you that needs no choice on your part. Place yourself in the middle of the stream of power and wisdom which flows into your life. Then, without effort, you are impelled to truth and to perfect contentment.

Several months ago, Alice told me, "I was lying in bed, ready to fall asleep, shortly after my evening meditation. I had a vision. It wasn't a dream, because I was not yet asleep and I was totally aware. I was in a dimly lit room. In one corner of the room was a doorway through which radiant light was coming. I saw the light as peaceful and beautiful, yet I was terrified to cross the doorway. I felt, though, it was now time to go through. As I stood in the doorway, enveloped by the light, there were two circles on the floor. I placed a foot in each circle. One circle contained powerlessness; the other, worthlessness. My entire life then passed before my eyes. I saw the fear that had been born from my illusion of powerlessness. Now that I was in the light, I saw powerlessness as completely illusory. I realized that I had never been powerless a single moment in my life. I realized I was an eternal being even when I was totally unaware of it. I forgave myself for all the decisions I'd made in fear, based in the illusion of powerlessness.

"I also observed the guilt and negative, hurtful decisions I'd made, based in the illusion of worthlessness," she went on. "I saw that this illusion was created when I was a young girl, about three years old. My whole life passed through my mind with the perspective that powerlessness and worthlessness had never been real. I was amazed to see how fear and guilt, which seemed so gigantic for so long, could be created from simple illusions that I adopted at such a young age. Now that I've been in the light, I have no fear of death. I know that I have been blessed to have this experience in my lifetime."

ESSENCE AND CHANGE

My patients who have glimpsed the power of their essence notice they have changed somehow. Their weariness vanishes. They begin to radiate a newfound joy and serenity. Often I or a family member note this change before the patient even becomes aware of it. One patient, who had been consumed with fear, begins to function more successfully in his work and is no longer afraid to take risks; another sees his power-hungry, insecure self lift and reveal a warm, compassionate soul. The depression of another patient over her son's death lifts as she glimpses some of life's universal truths.

Through the ESSENCE process, we discover a part of us that is nonjudgmental and free of resistance. Through this process, we can observe our faults, negative emotions, and fears. This state of objective awareness—allows us to see ourselves as if we were examining another person's life. This objectivity makes it easier not only to see but admit to our faults and our negative responses, since it is easier to see this in others than in ourselves. The ESSENCE process allows us to receive guidance, teaching, and direction from our essence and thus transcend the many conscious barriers to our higher self.

However, be aware that the mind will try to take credit for the peace, joy, and insight we achieve by touching our essence. Our mind thinks in its conditioned but conceited manner, "I arrived at this insight rationally. If I hold on to this way of thinking, I can and I must hold on to the good feelings I have also attained." The moment your mind thinks this, consciously or unconsciously, you have lost the experience. This experience and perspective can be lived, but only by being created anew *every day of your life*— not by trying to hold on to the memory of what you created yesterday.

We all know that some of us experience more pain in life than others. But we also know that all of us must go through tragedy, illness, and pain. We must experience, rather than avoid, these, because the pain of avoiding fear and sorrow is far greater than the pain of directly experiencing them. Whatever the accident, illness, or loss, ESSENCE imagery meditation allows us to be in touch with the lessons we must learn.

ESSENCE
Meditation:
Going Beyond Suffering

███

This ESSENCE meditation allows you to experience your suffering and clear the confusion that surrounds it. Begin this healing process by sitting quietly for two to three minutes with your eyes closed. Breathe deeply several times, inhaling into your abdomen as fully as you can, and then exhaling slowly all the air out of your lungs. Breathe in through your nose and out through your mouth. With each breath, repeat to yourself several of the following positive thoughts with the word *infinite* before them. For example, think of infinite healing, infinite truth, infinite light, and infinite peace. Visualize each breath being directed to a clear, blue mountain lake located in the upper part of your abdomen or solar plexus. Then simply observe your breathing for another two or three minutes without trying to control it.

1. EXPERIENCE

Experience and come to realize the suffering in your life.

Say to yourself, "I wish to experience the cause of my suffering that I see as originating outside myself." Ponder this and whatever realization and questions come up.

You might ask, "How much of my suffering originates outside myself? How much of my suffering originates within myself?" You might think about illness, loss of a loved one, or another unwanted occurrence.

Try to focus on only one or two of the things that are contributing most to your suffering. Then say to yourself, "I choose now to experience the feelings associated with my suffering." What do your feelings of suffering feel like inside your body? A pounding heart? A tense feeling in your stomach? Keep your attention on those areas as you experience these feelings.

Be aware of any questions that come up for you. You might ask, "What are my feelings associated with this unwanted reality? How am I suffering now?"

Experience the fear you have associated with this unwanted reality that you feel is the cause of your suffering. You might ask, "Why do I find this unwanted reality so frightening? What are the possible outcomes that I see arising out of this unwanted event?"

Feel the fear fully. You might fear that an illness represents ultimate failure and confirms your deeper fear that your life is meaningless and without lasting value. You might fear that the loss of a loved one means you will never know another day of happiness and cause you to doubt the existence of a higher truth or reality.

If you find the suffering or fear you are working on too uncomfortable, focus on others that are less troubling to work with first. You may need to work up to healing your greatest fears that engender suffering. If this is the case, say to yourself, "I know I will eventually have the confidence, guidance, and safety to heal all suffering in my life."

2. SEE

See and survey your reactions to what you view to be the cause of your suffering. Also notice any judgments you have about those causes as being bad or unjust. Your reaction may be one of anger that this unwanted occurrence happened to you. You may have reacted by feeling that your life has no meaning or by becoming depressed about illness or loss.

Say to yourself, "I realize that my reactions to my suffering and judgments about it originate in my mind and I am free to react differently and in a way that brings healing to my suffering."

Spend a few minutes thinking about this and allow your mind to ask any questions. You might ask, "Can my reactions to the causes of suffering in turn cause more suffering? What reactions are possible that would make me feel better, rather than worse, about the occurrence?"

3. SURRENDER

Surrender the cause of your suffering that you see as outside yourself to your essence. This means you must separate what you see as the cause of your suffering from your reactions and emotions about it.

Contemplate the following statement: "All my reactions to suffering are based on fear." Think about this carefully and then ponder the following: "Actions and reactions based on fear always engender more suffering."

You might ask, "How much of my suffering comes from an unwanted occurrence, and how much comes from my reactions to the occurrence?"

Now visualize the original cause of your suffering moving down and into your essence. Visualize your essence as a light above where you are sitting. Say to yourself, "I surrender to the light of my essence. I wish to learn any lessons or see any value that may be here for me."

As you contemplate this statement, allow any questions to come forth. You might ask, "What value or lesson could there be in occurrences that cause suffering? How can my essence bring healing to my suffering?"

4. EMPOWER

Empower and strengthen the healing of your suffering. Continue to visualize the light of your essence and picture it located above where you are aware of your suffering.

Say to yourself, "I ask my essence for the guidance, wisdom, and energy to heal my suffering, my fear associated with suffering, my reactions to this fear, and all the suffering this cycle engenders."

Spend a few minutes contemplating this, and be aware of any questions that come forth. You might ask, "What realization or wisdom could begin to lessen or heal my suffering? Where did this cycle of suffering, fear, and more suffering start, and how can it end?"

Say to yourself, "I am in reality greater than any illness, depression, or other unwanted reality. I am also greater than my fear and free to let it go at this moment. I realize that the suffering and fear have in no way ever hurt the reality of who I am."

5. NURTURE

Nurture this new realization. Sustain its existence and reality by saying to yourself, "I now feel and know the truth within my essence. I call on all the love, guidance, and wisdom within me to heal the suffering, fear, and negative emotions."

Draw on and visualize this light being sent to the suffering and to all the fear and emotions that surround it. Spend several minutes healing with this light.

6. CREATE

Create and behold a new reality in which the causes of your current suffering can exist, without your responses that engender more suffering.

Say to yourself, "My responses and reactions to unwanted occurrences lie within me, even though the unwanted occurrence might originate outside of myself. I am free to respond and react in ways that do not engender more fear and suffering."

Contemplate this statement, and allow any questions to come forth. You might ask, "What causes more suffering, the unwanted occurrence, or my thoughts and responses to this occurrence? Do I really have the power to respond differently? How would my life be different if I responded another way?"

7. EMBODY

Embody and integrate your realizations into your current reality.

Say to yourself, "When I am aware of my essence, suffering cannot be a reality."

Allow yourself to ask questions that come forth. You might ask, "What would my life be like without suffering?"

Further incorporate this light into your reality by saying, "I have glimpsed the real truth that is my essence. In the face of this, my suffering can lessen because I can choose how I respond and react to it. My ability and power to heal my suffering are far greater than I ever suspected."

Now slowly bring your awareness back to your body. Wait a minute or two before opening your eyes. You may wish to keep a journal to record any realizations that come to you now or later.

GOING BEYOND SUFFERING:
THE SEVEN STEPS WITH YOUR EYES CLOSED

Begin with the breathing exercise.

1. EXPERIENCE

Experience where in your body you feel your suffering. Feel its exact location, size, shape, color, and temperature. Visualize this as energy. Pick only one area of your body at a time.

2. SEE

Visualize the light of your essence located above the top of your head.

3. SURRENDER

Surrender your suffering to the higher power of your essence by visualizing its energy being released upwards into the light of your essence.

4. EMPOWER

Empower and strengthen this healing by recalling your essence. Again visualize the light of your essence flowing into the area you are working on.

5. NURTURE

Nurture the idea of a life free of suffering.

6. CREATE

Create a space for your higher power to continue to guide you by visualizing a channel through which the light of your essence can continue to flow in and the negativity you are working with can flow out.

7. EMBODY

Embody and externalize this healing by visualizing the light of your essence flowing into each cell of your body.

Path III:
Ending Melancholy

There are two kinds of sorrow and two kinds of joy. When a man broods over the misfortunes that have come upon him, when he cowers in a corner and despairs of help—that is a bad kind of sorrow, concerning which it is said: "The Divine Presence does not dwell in a place of dejection." The other kind is the honest grief of a man who knows what he lacks.

The same is true of joy. He who is devoid of inner substance and, in the midst of his empty pleasures, does not feel and does not try to fill his lack, is a fool. But he who is truly joyful is like a man whose house has burned down, who feels his need deep in his soul and begins to build anew. His heart rejoices over every stone that is laid.

—*Martin Buber,*
TEN RUNGS

The twentieth century, with all its progress and opportunity, has cultivated a virtual epidemic of melancholy. Depression affects a staggering number of people at some time in their lives. Even when things are going well, there is often a feeling that something is missing. For many of my patients, I have found that what is missing is an awareness of their soul or essence. From early childhood on, this awareness has been displaced by a need for success and conformity. People's idea of who they should be does not include an awareness of their essence, or of the value of solitude and time for contemplation.

As a society, we have little respect for our aging parents or for their wisdom borne of experience. We are no longer in awe of the sound of thunder or feel reverence for the changing of the seasons. We value buildings over forests, television sitcoms over books, and youth and health clubs over evenings at home with parents and grandparents. We are impressed by technological advances but are oblivious to the numerous subtle influences of nature. In turn, we have become burdened with melancholy.

How rare it can be for us to laugh without cause, to love for its own sake, to experience joy without expectations, or to open our heart without fear. Such laughter, love, joy, and openness can be rare parts of our lives, even though these emotions are intrinsic to who we really are. Instead, we have replaced these emotions with struggle and the pursuit of money, status, and success. This misplaced need for success and conformity at the expense of our essence leads to a burden of sorrow that is expressed as depression or melancholy.

EXPERIENCING MELANCHOLY

The ancient Taoist philosopher Chuang Tzu wrote:

> I cannot tell if what the world considers "happiness" is happiness or not. All I know is that when I consider the way they go about attaining it, I see them carried away headlong, grim and obsessed, in the general onrush of the human herd, unable to stop themselves or to change their direction. All the while they claim to be just on the point of attaining happiness.

Sorrow lurks in the shadow of each success and possession. We have all experienced melancholy in one way or another: through the loss of a loved one or a job, through a lack of fulfillment in our lives, or through a hopelessness about the future.

Psychiatry teaches that grief is a necessary and healthy emotional reaction to loss. Sorrow need not be judged as good or bad, nor should it be avoided. But each of us must see, without judgment or resistance, how sorrow has become a constant part of our lives. Chuang Tzu elaborated,

> Is there to be found on earth a fullness of joy, or is there no such thing? Is there some way to make life fully worth living, or is this impossible? If there is such a way, how do you go about finding it? What should you try to do? What should you seek to avoid? What should be the goal in which your activity comes to rest? What should you accept? What should you refuse to accept? What should you love? What should you hate?
>
> What the world values is money, reputation, long life, achievement. What it counts as joy is health and comfort of body, good food, fine clothes, beautiful things to look at, pleasant music to listen to.
>
> What it condemns is lack of money, a low social rank, a reputation for being no good, and an early death.
>
> What it considers misfortune is bodily discomfort and labor, no chance to get your fill of good food, not having good clothes to wear, having no way to amuse or delight the eye, no pleasant music to listen to. If people find that they are deprived of these things, they go into a panic or fall into despair. They are so concerned for their life that their anxiety makes life unbearable, even when they have the things they think they want. Their very concern for enjoyment makes them unhappy.
>
> The rich make life intolerable, driving themselves in order to get more and more money which they cannot really use. In so doing they are alienated from themselves, and exhaust themselves in their own service as though they were slaves of others.
>
> The ambitious run day and night in pursuit of honors, constantly in anguish about the success of their plans, dread-

ing the miscalculation that may wreck everything. Thus they
are alienated from themselves, exhausting their real life in
service of the shadow created by their insatiable hope.

The birth of a man is the birth of his sorrow.

We need to observe the sorrow in our lives in the context of
our desire for security, long life, health, and satisfaction. We need
to ask ourselves about the meaning of sorrow. Is it a reaction to
losing what our mind is attached to? Have we reduced the beauty
and light that surrounds us to petty, fragile images, destined for
destruction? Has sorrow diminished our purpose on earth, moved
us away from bringing love and light into the world and learning
the wonderful lessons of life, to holding a job that brings either
drudgery or the frustration that accompanies ambition?

NEEDS, DESIRE, AND AMBITION

What is the difference between our needs and our ambition? Our
bodies require the right nourishment and shelter, and when we
have them, our needs are fulfilled. Our essence also has simple
needs, although we have been largely unaware of those. Ambition
and desires, as opposed to needs, never belong to the present—
they are always in the future. Being driven by ambition is like
trying to find the pot of gold at the end of the rainbow. When
we were children, the point where the rainbow met the earth appeared close. But when we tried to find it, we found we could
walk forever and never get closer: what we saw was an illusion. It
is the same with our desires and ambitions. We have all desired to
have, or to be, many things, and yet when we had or became this
thing, we found that our desire or ambition had changed. We then
desired something more, something better or different. The distance between ourselves and the object of our *present* desire has
always remained the same, just as the distance between ourselves
and the point where the rainbow touches the earth has. The needs
of our bodies and our essence are simple and easily fulfilled,

whereas our desires and ambitions are complex and impossible ever to fulfill.

Desire and ambition have a connection with illness and healing. If desires consume too great a part of our lives and cause us to ignore the needs of our bodies and our essence, then they drain the energy necessary for us to function healthily. Most of us have been unable to take care of all our needs, because we have been focusing on living in the past or the future, not the present. Yet we still find our desires are not satisfied. This pattern will only leave us with less health and less fulfillment. But we can choose to live in the here and now, and healing is in the moment. There is no need—nor has there ever been—to ask for more.

You are here to live your truth, which is to experience fulfillment by listening to your essence. Others are here to live their own truth and find fulfillment by being in touch with their own inner nature. Many of your ambitions and desires result from the expectations others have for you. It is time to stop living up to others' expectations, and to stop expecting others to live up to yours.

EXPECTATIONS AND RESPECT

People become upset because their spouse, peers, teacher, or boss does not respect them. Everyone wants respect, but few understand what it really is. Respect is dignity born of understanding. When people understand you completely, they respect you and treat you with dignity. If they do not really understand who and what you are, they can never respect you. People falsely assume respect can be "earned." Earning respect from someone who doesn't understand you can only be done by denying the truth of who and what you are. After that, you have to conform to the illusion this person has about you. When you do this for hundreds of people over many years, you may experience great personal confusion.

Respect is born of understanding, and understanding cannot be earned. Somebody either does or doesn't understand you. The key is to remain true to yourself. Do not spend your life trying to conform to an illusion you have been taught to believe in. Rather, accept the fact that there will be some who do understand you, and many who don't.

To succeed in society and in the world of illusion, we often have to be insincere to our essence by lying to ourselves. When we care what others are thinking about us, we begin to live according to what they expect of us, not what is within our heart. And each time we aspire to live up to others' expectations, we lose the ability to live up to the best within ourselves. If we can finally let go of the need to fulfill others' expectations—and stop expecting anyone else to fulfill ours—we have taken a major step in living, by living in touch with our own essence. Whatever we believe, others do not suffer because we do not live up to their expectations: we only suffer because of what we create for ourselves, and others only suffer because of what they create for themselves. We may have more difficulty in life by refusing to live according to others' expectations, but that is far better than embarking on an unending cycle of continued separation from our essence, which results in living a lifetime of lies, detached from our soul.

In such a melancholic, detached state, we relinquish the bounty and beauty of the planet—its oceans, forests, and other sources of life—to the image of a lifeless rock. We forfeit joy, love, and laughter for ambition, jealousy, and violence, creating great sorrow for our essence. As the American pianist Arthur Rubinstein wrote, "Life holds so much—so much to be so happy about always. Most people ask for happiness on condition. Happiness can be felt only if you don't set conditions."

FREEDOM FROM SORROW

To free ourselves from sorrow, we must refrain from judging our sorrow as bad, for that will only cause us to resist it. And if we resist our sorrow, we deny its existence and thereby make it stronger. To be free of sorrow, we first must experience it, and become one with it by acknowledging its source. As with fear, we will eventually realize that we never knew sorrow; we only knew the avoidance of sorrow. We then experience the healing within us, for the sadness and tears that come with this realization are healing.

People experience a range of emotions as they embark on the ESSENCE process. Anger, sadness, fear, and doubt are but a few of the emotions that surround our essence like a wall, as noted earlier. These emotions must first be experienced before they can be healed and released. They have power over us now because they have been avoided, which has only strengthened them in our unconscious mind. This pattern of avoiding painful emotions and thus relinquishing them to our unconscious mind (where they increase in power) began when we were children. It has resulted in two of the greatest blocks to knowing our essence and its truth.

First, most of us made the following unconscious decision as a child: "I must totally avoid the experience of this pain, or it will destroy my life." Through this decision, we prevented our emotional selves or hearts from developing—like unused muscles—so that we cannot now experience any part of life as fully as we were meant to. Joy thus became for most of us a ridiculous, unobtainable dream, or a concept we could no longer relate to. Forgiveness became something that "nice people" were supposed to feel at times, rather than a consistent state of mind that we could develop to free us from most of our burdens.

The second ramification of our decision to relegate all painful emotions to our unconscious is that we allow these emotions to insidiously create intentions and beliefs that guide a large part of our lives. They can then attract circumstances and conditions that validate their reality. For instance, when a child repeatedly is yelled at or is told he or she is stupid or bad, a wound develops in the child's self-esteem. A child has no knowledge of how to heal this wound, so he or she represses it. However, it continues to fester; the deeper it is repressed, the harder it is to become aware of it and heal it.

Children may make many assumptions from such traumatic wounds. They may assume they are inherently bad or worthless. They may assume they are powerless. They may live with deep fear and guilt. We have thus created destructive beliefs, sorrows, and fears based on these unconscious emotions. They, in turn, keep us from learning the truth of who we are and why we are alive. In this way, we have given control of our thoughts and destiny largely to unconscious fears and beliefs. And more, these fears and beliefs have become intentions attracting conditions and circumstances that directly reflect those very intentions in our lives.

So how do we get past the sorrow we have created through this process? ESSENCE healing is a path through which we enrich our lives by embracing whatever fear, sadness, and sorrow remain with us. When we let go, just for a few minutes, of what blocks us from our essence, a part of us is healed. As the wall surrounding our essence begins to fall, we experience our power. The light within us begins to flow through each cell of our bodies, giving balance and healing. This healing flows to where it is most needed, as we temporarily let go of the blocks we have created.

The entire ESSENCE process first allows us to experience anything that keeps us from knowing the reality of who we are, and it then allows us to let go of that part of ourselves. Initially, you can experience the unlimited compassion and vastness of your essence only for a few minutes or even a few seconds. But such an experience, even if it lasts for only several seconds, can provide healing insight that can ease the sorrow and pain that have taken years to develop.

Mary: Cancer and Surrendering Attachment

■ Mary sought medical attention because she was having difficulty swallowing. She underwent a battery of tests that showed advanced cancer of the esophagus, which had already metastasized, or spread, to one lung. When she was referred to me, Mary confided that two years earlier she had lost her youngest child and only daughter, then age sixteen, in an automobile accident.

Unaware at the time of the significance of her words, she said, "I could never quite swallow this."

According to her husband, Mary had not been depressed, but she had never been the same since the death of their daughter.

She was a third-grade teacher, but after the accident she had requested and received a transfer to an administrative job. In her attempt to cut herself off from pain by avoiding anything that reminded her of her daughter, she began walling herself off from life itself. It was no longer just children that reminded Mary of her daughter, but anything that brought her joy. She had loved to swim and play tennis, but she no longer participated in either of these activities. Unconsciously, Mary had decided to die. I knew I could not force her to change this decision, nor was it my place to try. My function was to allow her to bring this desire to her consciousness, so that she could evaluate it in the context of her own inner truth.

Mary began working with the ESSENCE guided imagery process. I started her on a nutritional program, as well as chemotherapy. I also spent a great deal of time talking with her about her feelings and past traumas. She began to do some of the meditations. After several days, she told me that she kept having the feeling that she just wanted to be with her daughter. Then, one night, she had a dream.

"I came home from school with a headache, because the children had been particularly rowdy that day," she recounted. "I walked in and there were my three children and three of their friends sitting at the dining room table, each banging their knives and forks on the table for food. I saw the school principal talking to my husband in the other room, and I went in to ask for some help. As they turned toward me, I saw they had baby faces and were wearing diapers. I ran into the bedroom where my mother was crocheting, thinking that surely she could help me. She started crying, saying I had frightened her, and she wanted me to untangle a knot in her crochet string."

Mary saw how everyone in her life had become a child, and how identified with motherhood she had become. Subsequently, she was able to stand back, observe, and also separate herself from this attachment to the role of being a mother.

Mary realized the loss of her daughter wasn't the only thing she found "so hard to swallow"; she felt the same about facing the forced detachment from motherhood. Her strong self-image as a mother had dominated her life as both mother and teacher. Her daughter's death had forcibly removed her from the role of mother and caretaker, her major role throughout her married life. Her older children had left home for college several years before. This separation and loss of identity greatly contributed to her sorrow.

During a subsequent meditation, Mary experienced her daughter appearing to her as pure, white light.

"My mind became quiet and at peace," she told me. "I felt a sense of excitement, and before me was a pure light, white and shimmering. I knew it was my daughter. She said, 'Mom, there is only love, and love does not die. There is only one God, and we have never really been separate. Don't you know that God would never make a mistake with His child's life?' "

Following this, she tolerated her radiation and chemotherapy treatments with fewer and fewer side effects as she progressed with her spiritual development. She went on to attain a complete remission and lived her life as if she had never been ill. Mary realized that she loved her husband and two daughters far too much to want to leave them.

"It's what my daughter was telling me," she said to me. "I surrender today all the pain of yesterday, and I see only the essence within me. All around me, I see the beauty and perfection of nature."

We can see the same transcendence of pain into love in the apocryphal story of the eleventh-century Tibetan teacher Marpa, who learned of his son's sudden death. Marpa wept by himself as one of his disciples approached him and asked, "My teacher, you have instructed me in how suffering is an illusion and is created out of my attachment and clinging to the material world. If you, teacher, have so transcended resistance and attachment, then why do you weep?"

Marpa answered, "Yes, all in this world is illusion, and the death of a son is the greatest illusion of all."

Mary discovered that when she was able to surrender her rigid attachment to motherhood and the pain of losing her daughter, it did not represent failure. On the contrary, she created a space within her filled with the love and truth of her soul, and she discovered that her essence was even larger than her role as mother.

It is not our sorrow we must let go of, but our attachment to it. When we see that it is not all the things and issues in life that keep us in sorrow but our attachment to them, we can begin to release this attachment. When we can surrender to the flow of life like the change of seasons, we begin to understand and know our truth. We never know how long we will live or what events will befall us. Surely we will experience loss, but the suffering will only be magnified by our clinging and attachment to all that engenders fear in our lives.

The loss we feel when a child dies or when illness strikes cannot be minimized. We also feel sadness when we realize that we have hurt people, that we have carried anger for so long, and that we have missed out on life for so many years. But we can also realize that this was all because we were not aware of the truth, love, and light of our essence. We must allow this sadness and our tears to heal us. When we are living in truth, we know, like Mary, that a cherished person we lost may have completed his or her purpose on this earth. We know that to live fully, we must surrender our lives to our essence.

Roger: A Stomach Ulcer and the Transformation of Beliefs

■ Roger was a social work intern at a large New York medical center when he first came to see me. He complained of persistent indigestion and difficulty sleeping over the prior two months. He said he wanted to see me as his physician for a checkup, "because if anyone can find the cancer in me while it is early, it's you." I asked Roger why he was so sure that his symptoms represented cancer. He said he had been working the last six months on both the AIDS unit and the leukemia service at his hospital. He had seen a number of patients with whom he had developed close relationships die.

"So many patients I've tried to help are dying," Roger said. "The pain of knowing I'll never see these people again is making my whole life fall apart. Now that I'm feeling sick, I know it must be something serious."

After finding that Roger had developed a stomach ulcer, I placed him on a medication to help it heal. He said he was considering giving up his dream of becoming a therapist. I told him it was his decision whether to "play it safe" by pursuing a less intense career than counseling the sick and their families. I had Roger meditate on what, deep in his heart, he wanted to do with his life. I also had him focus on how fear was at the root of his current distress. I made recommendations for dietary changes, too. Lastly, I had Roger contemplate that he, as well as the patients he had been working with, all had an essence that could never be harmed by the fear, illness, and other adverse events that seemed so catastrophic to him at the time.

Roger thanked me for the guidance and said, "Maybe there is hope for me after all."

Roger's feelings of hope began immediately after his telling me what had been on his mind. This illustrates an important aspect of a healing doctor–patient relationship. This aspect is important in all healing, as well as in psychotherapy and confession. It is your human nature to attract healing the moment you can honestly share who you are, with openness and trust, to your doctor, therapist, or clergyperson. It was during this moment that Roger did not need to appear less afraid than he really was. For a moment, he did not have to live a lie. This is why all doctor–patient relationships must have the safety and trust necessary for patients to be able to speak openly and honestly.

I saw Roger the following week. He told me his indigestion had resolved and he was sleeping normally again. In time, he realized he had gone into social work and counseling not just to make a living but to help other people.

"My fears are the issue here," he said. "My fear of sickness and death has resulted from my identification with only my body, ambitions, and worries. It was neglect of my essence that allowed my fear to lead me to believe that any ache or pain signaled an end to all that I feared I was. Once I let my fear go for a few minutes, I discovered the peace that came with awareness of my reality and my truth. I now realize that my attachment to fear can only lead me to suffer."

Roger saw that the illusion and fear that had guided his life could be transformed through perspective and acceptance. He realized this through the ESSENCE process, in which he received healing insight. He felt deep compassion for, and acceptance of, his body, which could become ill and would eventually die. The insight provided by this feeling of compassion then transformed his thoughts and his life. He realized that his fear of his own mortality separated him from his essence, and from his patients as well. He could safely accept his physical reality, and this also allowed him to convey this acceptance to his patients, as they felt the healing radiating from his essence. Roger thus realized how his fear had led to his destructive beliefs, which eventually could have led to far more serious consequences than a stomach ulcer.

If you believe, as Roger did initially, that you cannot change, that the world is a threatening place, and that your destiny in life is for everything "to fall apart," then you will experience just that. All your beliefs either unconsciously reflect or become your intentions. Roger was fortunate enough to see this reality and transform his beliefs, as well as his unconscious intentions, before they ruined his life.

If you truly believe that you can let go of all despair, hopelessness, and guilt—and also begin to believe, as you experience your essence, that your life can be filled with abundance, health, and joy—you can begin to make this the reality of your life.

Whenever you become harried, worried, or anxious, you have made the unconscious choice that what is outside (in the world) is more important than what is inside (in your heart). You have also made the choice that doubt is more important than trust.

Doubt has become a habit for most of us. Bad habits, like cancers, can multiply out of control if not checked. This is why meditation is so important. When you can make a habit of trusting your essence, even when doubt is present, an inner peace can be maintained throughout adversity. It is all a matter of living in the moment and being conscious of what is internal and what is external. Then you may choose to trust what is inside rather than doubt what is outside. You can doubt only when your awareness is in the past or the future. When your awareness is in the moment, no matter what you are doing becomes a meditation in itself. That is why now—this very moment—is synonymous with eternity. When you are aware of your essence, you can always only be in the moment. Thus, your essence knows *only* eternity, because the moment is eternity.

By maintaining the intention to experience your essence and its truth, you bring forth your ability to experience healing, abundance, and a deep sense of your own worth in all situations. When you begin to see your obstacles and misconceptions as opportunities for growth, you begin to understand the Buddhist saying, "The greater the hindrance, the greater the enlightenment." The depression that can arise from adversity, illness, and loss can thus be seen as stepping-stones along your own path for healing.

ESSENCE
Meditation:
Ending Melancholy

This is a seven-step process for ESSENCE healing of your sadness, sorrow, or depression. Sorrow can be associated with a number of other painful emotions such as loneliness and despair.

Sit comfortably on a couch or chair in a quiet place with your eyes closed for two or three minutes. Breathe deeply several times, inhaling into your abdomen as fully as you can. Slowly exhale all the air from your lungs. Breathe in through your nose and out through your mouth. With each breath, repeat to yourself several of the following positive thoughts with the word *infinite* before them. For example, think of infinite healing, infinite truth, infinite light, and infinite peace. Visualize each breath being directed to a clear, blue mountain lake located in the upper part of your abdomen or solar plexus. Then simply take two to three minutes observing each breath without trying to control it.

1. EXPERIENCE

Experience and feel the sorrow in your life.

Take a minute to relax and then say to yourself, "I wish to feel my sorrow." Pay attention to your body. How does your sorrow feel? What do you feel in your stomach? Do you feel sorrow in your heart? For now, select only one area where there is sorrow to work on.

Say to yourself, "I wish to experience what areas in my life are most associated with sorrow."

Allow any questions to come forth. You might ask, "Does my sorrow originate outside of me? Is my feeling of sorrow different and separate from my feeling of fear?" Spend a few minutes experiencing and contemplating whatever questions arise.

2. SEE

See and survey the results of sorrow in your life.

Say to yourself, "I see all the other emotions associated with my sorrow." As you see these, do not delve further into them right now.

Be aware of any questions that arise. You might ask, "What are the results of sorrow in my life? Does my sorrow engender anything that serves me in a positive way?"

Say to yourself, "I have given birth to my sorrow by forgetting my essence. What I have created, I can transform." Feel your power to accomplish this transformation.

As you contemplate this, be aware of any questions that come up for you, such as, "How did I create my sorrow? If forgetting my essence created sorrow, what will remembering bring?"

Say to yourself, "I now allow myself to see my sorrow and my emotions surrounding my sorrow, so that they can be healed."

3. SURRENDER

Surrender to your essence the pain, loneliness, and sadness that arise as you experience your sorrow. As you surrender these, feel the pain, loneliness, and sadness as fully as you can. The act of surrendering these painful feelings to your essence creates a safety that may allow you to experience them truly for the first time.

Say to yourself, "I give myself the freedom to feel and fully experience my sorrow. I have no need to fight it any longer, because now is the time for healing."

Contemplate this for several minutes and be aware of any questions that come up. You might ask, "How can surrender bring healing? What will it feel like to stop resisting this?"

4. EMPOWER

Empower and strengthen this healing process.

Say to yourself, "It is my intention to heal my sorrow and, in its place, to know love, harmony, and joy."

Ponder this and allow any questions to emerge. You might ask, "What would replace my sorrow if it was no longer in my life?"

Part of empowering your intention is seeing your need to resist and avoid your sorrow. Say to yourself, "I have the power and safety in my essence to experience and heal rather than continue to avoid my sorrow."

Contemplate this and see what questions come up for you. You might ask, "If avoidance of sorrow feels like this, what will healing of it feel like?"

5. NURTURE

Nurture and cultivate your realizations and experience of the power within your essence.

Say to yourself, "My sorrow was born out of forgetting, and now it is time to remember."

Contemplate this and see what questions come forth. You might ask, "Can sorrow exist in the same mind that really knows the truth of its soul?"

Visualize the power of your essence aligned with that of the universe. With all the strength of your will, say to yourself, "I have unlimited power to have what is my birthright: joy, peace, and harmony that is free from my sorrow. I deserve this and ask all the energies of my higher self to bring this into my life."

Spend a few minutes with these thoughts. Be open to any questions that come forth. You might ask, "How is it I never knew such power before? How could I not have seen such beauty when it was within me all along?"

6. CREATE

Create a vision of your life free from sorrow. Ask yourself what attachments, lifestyle choices, and attitudes in your life engender sorrow. Feel your resistance to letting go of these causes.

Say to yourself, "I do not need sorrow in my life. I choose to let go of the causes of sorrow in my life and embrace the power of my essence." Contemplate this for several minutes.

Be aware of any questions that arise. You might ask, "Am I willing to free myself from my attachments to the causes of my sorrow? If I do not deserve sorrow, what do I deserve?"

7. EMBODY

Embody and actualize this vision by deeply feeling your desire and your will to let go of the causes of sorrow in your life. It is not enough to think this—you must really feel it. Muster all your will, determination, and desire to be free of sorrow in your life.

Say to yourself, "I choose to have what I know I deserve: peace, harmony, and freedom from my sorrow." When you say that with will and determination, you initiate a whole creative process that will manifest this reality in your life.

Sit with this thought for a few minutes before bringing your awareness back to your body. Then sit quietly a minute or two more before opening your eyes. You may now wish to record any realizations or questions in a journal. You may proceed to the ESSENCE Guided Imagery meditation, or take a break and do this at a later time.

ENDING MELANCHOLY:
THE SEVEN STEPS WITH YOUR EYES CLOSED

Begin with the breathing exercise.

1. EXPERIENCE

Experience where in your body you feel your sadness. Feel its exact location, size, shape, color, and temperature. Visualize this as energy. Pick only one area of your body at a time.

2. SEE

Visualize the light of your essence located above the top of your head.

3. SURRENDER

Surrender your sadness to the higher power of your essence by visualizing its energy being released upwards into the light of your essence.

4. EMPOWER

Empower and strengthen this healing by recalling your essence. Again visualize the light of your essence flowing into the area you are working on.

5. NURTURE

Nurture the idea of a life free of sadness or melancholy.

6. CREATE

Create a space for your higher power to continue to guide you by visualizing a channel through which the light of your essence can flow in and the negativity you are working with can flow out.

7. EMBODY

Embody and externalize this healing by visualizing the light of your essence flowing into each cell of your body.

Path IV:
Creating Hope

"Hope" is the thing with feathers—
That perches in the soul—
And sings the tune without the words—
And never stops—at all—
            —*Emily Dickinson*,
            No. 254, st. 1

Hope is the light that emanates from the soul. Hope can lead us to know truth and wisdom. Hope provides a framework for healing to begin.

Creating a healing attitude and outlook requires that we begin to notice and constantly question our own thoughts. We all carry on an almost constant internal conversation. This chain of thoughts rarely stops during our waking hours. It offers a commentary on how our lives should be, and judgments about ourselves and others. Our thoughts cause us to react with fear about present illusions and anticipated events. We create theories and criticisms about the meanings of our traumas and misfortunes.

If our mind continues to explain all the events, setbacks, and tragedies in the way it has been taught since childhood, we fall back into a pattern of fear, illusion, and, eventually, hopelessness. To live in truth, we must constantly question the internal dialogue within our own mind. Finding the truth and purpose unique to our own essence only partially enables us to experience the joy that is our birthright. We must also have the courage and wisdom to know how to *live* that truth. Wisdom is seeing the world through the eyes of the soul; hope is explaining the world from the viewpoint of the soul.

Discovering our essence does not mean that life will no longer include unwanted events, setbacks, and even tragedies. But when we give up the need to judge our setbacks as bad, we can evolve. With wisdom, we can talk to ourselves about unwanted events from the viewpoint of our essence. This may be an entirely new form of internal conversation for us—one that results in a profound change in attitude.

As the other ESSENCE paths have shown us, fear, worry, and depression are based on negative thoughts, the avoidance of which causes our painful feelings. We avoid them because we think they have power. Thoughts cannot hurt us, but we think that they can, so we give them power that in reality they don't have. When our thoughts are negative and destructive in this way, they are out of alignment with who we really are. This is why they make us feel depressed, fearful, or ashamed. However, they can be replaced with thoughts based on our essence.

The surest way for us to begin thinking in alignment with our essence is to question the origin of each of our thoughts. We need to ask ourselves whether a certain thought associated with feelings of fear or anxiety has any inherent power or reality, or whether it is just a thought that can be replaced with another based on the reality of who we are. The ESSENCE process allows us to see how *we* have empowered the thoughts that make us feel miserable, depressed, or even sick. Many of us falsely think that our thoughts about ourselves are actually us. Learning that our thoughts in and of themselves *have no power* over us allows us to see and embrace life fully, rather than live as a prisoner of our old, destructive thought patterns.

Beliefs are not necessarily truths. A patient once said to me, "I failed in my life, and now that I'm sick, I feel it is just a punishment for all these failures." I've heard many such statements from patients. Not only are these conclusions false, but they are the self-fulfilling product of faulty thinking produced by a number of previous misfortunes: overly critical parents, childhood loss, or a loved one's illness. Because we sometimes think as this patient did, we accept such thoughts as gospel truth. However, they are nothing more than beliefs, and believing something does not make it true.

EXAMINE YOUR BELIEFS ABOUT YOURSELF

You need to begin to question your explanations of life's events from the viewpoint and truth of your essence. Whenever your beliefs become obvious to you, question them *immediately* from the viewpoint of your essence. In your mind or on paper, think through a dialogue beween parts of yourself. Take for example the following beliefs about adversity, and the ways your essence can heal these fears:

YOUR FEAR: This can make my life fall apart.
YOUR ESSENCE: I surrender to the reality that nothing in this world was meant to last forever. I surrender to the light of my essence.
YOUR FEAR: This can only lead to a terrible outcome.
YOUR ESSENCE: I cannot foresee all of the turns life can take, but I have overcome adversity in the past, and I can do it again.
YOUR FEAR: My life can never be the same, now that this has happened.
YOUR ESSENCE: My life is never the same from one day to the next. It is different today than it was yesterday, and tomorrow it will be different as well. How boring it would be to live a stagnant life without change.
YOUR FEAR: What if this horrible thing does happen someday? I just couldn't deal with it.
YOUR ESSENCE: I will not dwell on this horrible occurrence. I could just as well dwell on a thousand others that I haven't yet

thought of. My life has uncertainty because I was not *meant* to know the future. This is a gift that gives my life richness, not a curse that makes my life miserable.

Personalize each of the preceding statements with occurrences in your own life. Notice your experience and reactions to each statement. Can you see then how having thousands of thoughts based on fear each day can make you feel? Can you see how, if all your thoughts were based on essence, your life could be healed?

When you are afraid, worried, or depressed about a situation, you are not experiencing it from the viewpoint of who you really are. Any situation, when experienced and explained by your essence, immediately becomes less negative because it is accepted, and it is accepted because your essence knows that no situation can ever hurt the reality of who you are. Life, when experienced from your essence, becomes quite simple as you free yourself from attachment to fear. The richness of a star-filled sky, the company of those you love, and the feeling of peace that accompanies surrender become far more important than the threatening illusions that have given rise to your fear.

Nearly always, we have questions: Does my belief that I am a failure, that I am unlovable, or that I am inadequate carry any reality in the context of the reality of who I am based on my essence? From the viewpont of my soul, is there any validity to my negative beliefs that I am a failure or unlovable? As you consider such questions, standing back from your belief and immediately questioning it allows you to distance yourself from it long enough to verify its truth. Feel free to dispute your automatic thoughts and beliefs. The first step in living your truth is to notice and be aware of these seemingly reflexive explanations and beliefs. The second is to allow these explanations and beliefs to fall by the wayside as the truth and light of your essence shine through them.

Jim: Colon Cancer and a Questioning of Assumptions

▪ Jim, a successful accountant, had colon cancer that had spread to his liver, which was swollen and very painful. In his second week of chemotherapy, he told me, "My cancer is far too advanced for this chemotherapy to have any effect."

I worked with him through counseling, diet, nutritional support, and chemotherapy and asked him to examine these assumptions from another point of view. I also asked him how this pattern of thinking began and may have shaped his life, as well as his view of himself and the world. His answer was, "Numbers are numbers and the statistics don't look good."

On his visit one week later, he stated that during an ESSENCE Guided Imagery meditation he realized that the numbers with which he had been so concerned during his whole career were a shield from both his fears and the truth. He had begun to question his belief that he was no different from the numbers in a textbook, and also to question the implications of such thinking. The main implication, he found, was to be separated not only from vitality and joy, but from any creative possibilities.

"If everything in life is cut and dried and calculated in advance, what's the point in even being here?" Jim asked. To him, the answer was obvious: there was no point. But he saw during subsequent counseling how he used numbers and logic as a way to compensate for several childhood traumas and overly critical parents. When he caught himself thinking that a painful death was the only logical conclusion to having cancer, he questioned the truth of this. His reponse was a question: "Do I really think I can know all of the possibilities the universe has given to the essence within me?"

The prayer he had been taught as a child now gave him great strength. "The power of God is within me. The grace of God surrounds me." Jim went on to have a partial remission with complete resolution of his pain, and he is back at work almost a year after his diagnosis.

As Jim learned, we must be willing not only to question our thoughts but also to argue with ourselves. Is our belief false? Is it destructive? Does it allow us to live to the truth of our essence? A little healing happens with each question we raise, because we are beginning to allow truth to come into our reality. The rhetorical questions I use in ESSENCE Guided Imagery, as described throughout this book, are a way of focusing our mind to ask the questions that will lead us to this truth.

Jim saw how he explained adversity by reducing it to a numerical equation with only one—usually negative—solution or conclusion. He found that questioning this explanation opened a whole realm of possibilities for him to explore. He knew that cancer could bring death and pain. However, it could and did bring spiritual growth, healing, and discovery of joy among his family and friends. He also discovered by no longer confining the universe to his own pad and pencil that he himself had great power. Once he found that the world was not a fearful place, he no longer walled himself off from it. He had made a realization about which the French writer Albert Camus once said, "In the midst of winter, I finally learned that there was in me an invincible summer."

Sheila: Breast Cancer and the Acceptance of Love

■ Sheila came under my care six months ago. She was thirty-seven years old and had been diagnosed a year earlier with a very aggressive form of breast cancer. From another doctor, she had received intensive chemotherapy and radiation and had had one breast surgically removed. The side effects of the chemotherapy, radiation, and surgery were, in her words, "worse than the doctors even expected." She had a relapse of cancer in her bones and liver.

I could sense the tremendous sadness in her. I also sensed her resistance to receiving any of the treatments she already had, as well as any further therapy. Her father had died of a brain tumor when she was seven years old. She said, "I never quite got my feet on the ground since then."

During an ESSENCE Guided Imagery meditation, Sheila, in a very moving realization, said she felt the presence of her father. She stated that he wanted her to know he was quite happy on a nonphysical plane, and to be assured he had never left her, but only changed form. She recalled instances in her life in which she now felt that he had been present and had given her light and assistance, even though she had not been aware of it at the time. She realized that she had been carrying anger at her father for abandoning her and had blamed the loneliness she felt as a child on her mother. Her mother had had to work two jobs to support Sheila, so she had rarely been around to help Sheila with homework or to attend school functions.

"I was also ashamed of her," Sheila admitted to me. "She worked as a waitress at a local restaurant in the evenings and cleaned houses during the day. I feel so guilty. She did every-thing she could for me and never thought about herself. How could I have been ashamed of my mother?"

Sheila cried at the pain she had caused her mother and flew home to Pittsburgh to share this with her. "I told her that I loved her. I told her that I respected her for her dedication to me. We both cried."

Sheila continued to heal her confusion and began to forgive herself. She saw how her anger and embarrassment were the only ways that, as a young girl, she could work out the tragedy in her life. For years, Sheila had also had difficulty in finding a man with whom she could have a meaningful relationship. She had always assumed it was because "none were willing to make a commitment." But she came to realize that the relationships in her life had failed largely because of the self-fulfilling, faulty ideas that she had developed about men, commitment, and love. Over the next few months, Sheila discovered and healed much of her pain. Her own fears of death, illness, and life dropped away. She had few side effects from the chemotherapy and con-tinues to regain her health.

As a child, Sheila had adopted two faulty attitudes about life. First, she assumed that happiness and pleasure were impossible, but loss, fear, and pain were synonymous with reality. This led to a second assumption: to create happiness and joy (since she believed this could only be done through fantasy or dreams), she needed to escape from the reality of life. This left her no choice but to withdraw from meaningful relationships, never to risk embarking on creative endeavors, and never to pursue anything that gave her pleasure. What Sheila discovered was that life includes not only loss but also creation, and it consists of not only emotional pain but also pleasure. Relationships did not result in only rejection but love and warmth too. Each time she glimpsed her essence, her confusion lessened.

TRANSFORMATION AND DISCOVERY

We all have feelings of discouragement and helplessness. However, our ability to transform our internal dialogue can make the difference between despair and joy. Failure to accomplish this transformation does not mean there is a lack of will or ability. But it does imply that we do not yet see the urgency and absolute importance of doing so. When we do see it, transformation will be accomplished with the determination of a drowning person trying to reach air, or of someone dying of thirst in a desert trying to find water.

If your reaction to adversity is, "It's all over—I can't handle this one," then you will give up and be separated from the light of your essence. Instead, you can see adversity and unwanted events as challenges that can teach you necessary lessons. Adversity can bring you wisdom that you might not otherwise attain. The mind, as we have seen, first tries to explain adversity in conditioned ways, judging it as bad and resisting it. But by taking control of your thoughts and by questioning and challenging your initial reactions, you can prevent negative, destructive attitudes about life and allow hope to guide your explanations.

Hope allows your outlook to be more aligned with your essence.

You can replace your negative, destructive conclusions and explanations about life with more constructive, positive ones that emanate from your essence. You will no longer need to "build" self-confidence; you will naturally begin to trust in your own higher power. Conceit will also be replaced with humility, for as you move toward your essence, you let go of the need to judge, criticize, and condemn yourself and others. You learn to trust your heart, rather than struggle with the world.

Sarah: Ovarian Cancer and Anger

▌Sarah came to see me for the first time just over a year ago. Recently diagnosed with advanced ovarian cancer, she had undergone a hysterectomy and removal of her ovaries several weeks before seeing me. The disease had already spread to her liver and one lung, and she was very angry about the circumstances that had befallen her.

"I haven't had such an easy life," she told me on her first visit. "It isn't fair that this happened to me. My husband and children try to be supportive, but they don't have to go through this. I do. Everything bad always seems to happen to me."

I asked her what other bad things in her life she was referring to.

"I was driving late one night with my sister on a country road when I was sixteen," Sarah answered. "We'd had a couple of beers and were headed home. I always put on my seat belt; Sally rarely did. I was speeding and suddenly saw a pickup truck crossing the road as I was driving up a hill. There was no way I could stop in time. Sally was killed instantly. I was banged up pretty bad, but I lived."

I noticed an amazing lack of sadness as Sarah related this to me.

She said she had been in psychotherapy for ten years following her sister's death. "My parents never said it, but of course it was my fault. I understand it all. I have deep-seated guilt about something I can't change. It only cost me $25,000 to learn that."

Sarah began chemotherapy and nutritional support for her cancer, as well as ESSENCE Guided Imagery meditations and counseling sessions with me. She had several side effects from the chemotherapy, including hair loss and severe nausea.

Her daughter and husband came with her on one of her visits. In their presence, she said, "I have a confession to make. I know I've tried to blame every single thing that has happened to me over the years on the two of you. At times, it may have been subtle, but I always knew I was doing it. I'm really sorry."

For the first time, I witnessed the tremendous sadness inside Sarah. I asked her if, during her meditations, she could get more in touch with the guilt she was carrying around. On her next visit, she told me, "I really did experience my guilt. It feels like a constricting vice around my shoulders and heart, with a lead weight attached to it. I also feel I'm about to find a way to remove it."

Sarah continued with the chemotherapy. In two months, she was in a complete clinical remission, with a normal CAT scan and normal tumor markers (a blood test for ovarian cancer). She continued with the ESSENCE process.

On a subsequent visit, she told me, "I now see what I have been doing to myself through my feelings and thoughts since my sister's death. I loved her so much, and I still really miss her. I know I can't have her back, but I also know in some way we will be together again. I don't want to hurt myself or my family ever again out of my guilt."

For the first time, Sarah realized the destructive path she had been on. "I see what I have done to others and myself while seeking a way to handle my guilt. I was trying to resolve my guilt by punishing myself and those around me. I can't believe the years of effort I've expended trying to resolve something that cannot be resolved through effort. I can't begin to fathom all the time I've spent trying to understand something that can't be reasoned away. I can't believe the hurt I've caused, by punishing my family and myself for something punishment could never relieve. I now know where to begin: by forgiving the sixteen-year-old girl within me who has always done the best she could. I must also find forgiveness for all that I've done out of my faulty perception that I had to punish and be punished."

Sarah understood that forgiveness is a consistent state of mind rather than an act regarding a single event. She also realized the difference between understanding with her mind and understanding with her heart. The understanding and perspective that she obtained with her heart is what I call healing insight, which leads to a release of the fears, shame, and guilt we impose on ourselves. When we touch our essence, as Sarah did, a fundamental gift such as forgiveness is imparted to us.

Sarah remains in complete remission. She had a second surgical procedure six months ago to perform biopsies, which confirmed that the remission was stable.

Healing insight and perspective are logical and sane when thought about with our rational mind, although these can never be arrived at or created through logic alone. Healing insight is not the result of thinking a certain way, reasoning, or reciting positive affirmations; it is bestowed by our essence and experienced in the quiet of our own heart. Healing insight is always initially experienced as compassion, free of thought. Only then does it lend itself to our mind and thoughts.

Sarah's life had taken a destructive path after she had chosen to withdraw from the pain she had experienced over her sister's death. This withdrawal had only exacerbated her subconscious guilt. Sarah, like many of us, had made the unconscious decision, "I must never feel my sadness or guilt if I wish to prevent the pain from destroying my life." Most of us have made many similar unconscious decisions as children. Unhappy circumstances and events occur in every child's life: disappointment, failure to win a parent's approval, pain, and discomfort. The more we relegate the natural pain and disappointment associated with unwanted events to our unconscious, the more we wall off our ability to experience our essence, and thus life itself. By avoiding the experience of pain, we also inhibit our ability to experience the richness of life, and then we wonder why the experience of happiness always seems so elusive. Such withdrawal from experiencing painful emotions leads to the inhibition of our emotional selves. If we lose the ability to feel, how can we then expect to create the love, joy, and harmonious relationships we long for? We can't have it both ways. If we choose to protect ourselves from our emotions, we cannot open ourselves to life.

The decision to protect ourselves in this manner is a choice for safety in a world of illusion—a choice that provides not safety but isolation and an emotionally constricted existence. It results in a pessimistic outlook, through which we blame lack of love and fulfillment on bad luck, bad parents, or bad circumstances. We must discover, like Sarah, that we caused this state of pessimism and isolation, and that we can change it by discovering our essence. After we do so, our lives take on a new energy and a newfound intuition based on inner power and a deep sense of our own adequacy. Of course, we will stumble from time to time, falling into old patterns and old explanations. But if we make each stumbling block another stepping-stone in the development of new attitudes and explanations, the transformation of our lives must occur.

Forgiveness is an important state of mind on the path to healing. Forgiveness, like surrender, must be experienced, not just thought about. Forgiveness and surrender allow us to gently let go of whatever keeps us from knowing the truth in our heart. When we are identified with guilt, fear, or sorrow, it seems impossible to simply let them go. This is why we must first experience them and allow them to be. We then stop avoiding them, judging them, and resisting them. When we can first be with what it is that we've been avoiding, we have the potential to let it go. Thus, we can understand our lives from a perspective that now engenders hope rather than fear and guilt.

Creating forgiveness each day allows us to be attuned to what truth lies within our essence. Forgiveness is a state of mind that allows us to accept what is imperfect in ourselves and the world, rather than continue to resist it, and thus block out any chance for true change. What we resist will persist; what we accept can transform.

When you can see your imperfections, guilt, and past with compassion, you begin to understand the teaching of the Buddha: If you searched the entire world, you would find no one more deserving of love than yourself. When you understand your innate right to experience this love and light, there can no longer be any doubt that hope exists.

ESSENCE
Meditation: Creating Hope

This seven-step ESSENCE Guided Imagery and meditation is designed to assist you in seeing how your destructive, negative explanations (many of which are unconscious) contribute to your suffering. You may ask, "Why would I wish to change my explanations to myself about my life?" To answer this, simply see how explanations based on fear can only cause more pain and suffering. Explanations originate in your thoughts, however, and can be changed. A change of these explanations can engender hope where there was despair, and courage where there was fear. Remember, no matter how negative your attitude is, it does not alter the fact that healing and transformation are available to you by looking to your essence. The capacity to develop hope is one of the most important aspects of your ability to bring healing into your life. Hope springs forth from trust in your essence. This trust is essential in the healing process.

Begin by sitting on a couch or chair in a quiet room. Take several deep breaths. Slowly inhale deeply into the upper part of your abdomen. Then exhale slowly as completely as you can. Breathe in through your nose and out through your mouth. With each breath, repeat to yourself several of the following positive thoughts with the word *infinite* before them. For example, think of infinite healing, infinite truth, infinite light, and infinite peace. Visualize each breath being directed to a clear, blue mountain lake located in the upper part of your abdomen or solar plexus. Then take another two or three minutes to observe your breathing without trying to control it.

1. EXPERIENCE

Experience how you explain to yourself illness or another unwanted occurrence in your life. Experience how these explanations make you feel when you think about them.

Say to yourself, "My explanations about [whatever you're focusing on] originate within me, even though I see this occurrence as having originated outside myself."

Contemplate this for a few moments and be aware of any questions that come up. You might ask, "How do my explanations make me feel? What is the difference between how this occurrence makes me feel and how my explanations of it make me feel?"

Spend a few minutes thinking about the conclusions you have drawn about the unwanted event or illness. Experience how you have explained why it happened and what outcomes you have seen as likely.

Say to yourself, "I wish to experience what this occurrence or illness means."

Ponder this statement and notice what questions come up. You might ask, "Does this have any inherent meaning, or only that which I give it? Who decided what meaning this should have for me?"

2. SEE

See how you can choose different, more constructive explanations aligned with your essence.

Say to yourself, "I am free to choose what I believe about this unwanted reality and my life. I can explain this and draw conclusions about it in a way that can bring hope and healing rather than despair and fear."

Spend a few minutes contemplating this and allow any questions to come forth. You might ask, "What other beliefs and explanations are possible about this unwanted reality? Do I have any current beliefs that bring me hope and healing?"

Say to yourself, "My outlook and explanations, which seem to be concrete and permanent, are actually nothing more than thoughts that can be changed."

Think about this and be aware of any questions that arise. You might ask, "Is my outlook on life just a simple thought? Can my thoughts be changed?"

3. SURRENDER

Surrender your negative explanations and outlook to your essence. Visualize your essence as a light radiating warmth and serenity above where your awareness is now. Slowly picture your awareness moving into this light.

Say to yourself, "I choose to heal my attitude and outlook, based on fear, despair, and sadness, with the unlimited love and energy of my essence. I surrender to this healing light and send it throughout my mind and thoughts." Spend a few minutes in this light with these thoughts.

What questions come to you? You may ask, "What are my new explanations for what has happened? What is my new attitude?" As you think about your own questions, stay focused on your intention to heal your outlook.

4. EMPOWER

Empower your new outlook and hope. Do this by feeling total trust in your essence to replace your explanations and conclusions based on fear and despair with those based on truth and harmony.

Say to yourself, "My outlook, attitude, and explanations are my reality now, but they are not based on truth. I realize this is a temporary reality, and I wish to create a new reality based within my essence. I trust in my power to transform my conclusions, outlook, and attitudes, which do not please or serve me well."

Spend several minutes allowing the healed explanations, attitudes, and outlook to flow into your consciousness. See how much more positive they are compared to the old ones and how much better they make you feel.

5. NURTURE

Nurture and cultivate these new explanations by saying to yourself, "While I may not be able to control all events and circumstances in my life, I can control my attitudes, explanations, and conclusions about them. No matter what happens, I choose to think about my life with constructive thoughts and heal it with all the resources available to my essence." Spend a few minutes with these thoughts.

Be aware of any questions that come up. You may ask, "When have I changed my attitude before? What conclusions have I made that cause me to have a dreary outlook on life?"

6. CREATE

Create a space for further healing of any negative attitudes or outlooks you still feel you have.

Say to yourself, "I have not healed all of my negative explanations and conclusions about this experience. However, this does not mean I have failed. It means my working on this area will continue as long as I continue to let go of fear. I have created my fear, and as I have healed other fears, I can and will heal this also." Spend a few minutes with these thoughts.

Allow any questions or realizations to come forth. You may ask, "Can I now have a space where I can heal my fears and negative attitudes? Can I come to this space in the future to ask what a negative occurrence in life means?"

7. EMBODY

Embody and integrate these realizations into your awareness and being.

Say to yourself, "When my explanations and conclusions move me toward health, harmony, and fulfillment, they are being used as intended by my essence. When they are based in fear, they engender more fear. I ask to have the wisdom to choose the path of healing."

Spend a few minutes with these thoughts, and allow any questions and realizations to come forth. You might ask, "Where does the path of healing lead? What path am I currently on?"

Now, slowly transfer your awareness back to your body. Take a couple of slow, deep breaths and sit for a few minutes before opening your eyes.

It is particularly helpful to keep a journal to write down your thoughts and realizations after completing this ESSENCE Guided Imagery. Remember, the creative process you stimulate with the process of ESSENCE healing will bring healing from outside yourself as well. Be attuned to events, people you meet, and books you come across "by accident" that can facilitate your healing and spiritual growth.

CREATING HOPE:
THE SEVEN STEPS WITH YOUR EYES CLOSED

Begin with the breathing exercise.

1. EXPERIENCE
Experience where in your body you feel your negative outlook or hopelessness about any aspect of your life. Feel its exact location, size, shape, color, and temperature. Visualize this as energy. Pick only one area of your body at a time.

2. SEE
Visualize the light of your essence located above the top of your head.

3. SURRENDER
Surrender your negative outlook to the higher power of your essence by visualizing its energy being released upwards into the light of your essence.

4. EMPOWER
Empower and strengthen this healing by recalling your essence. Again visualize the light of your essence flowing into the area you are working on.

5. NURTURE
Nurture the idea of a life free of negative outlooks.

6. CREATE
Create a space for your higher power to continue to guide you by visualizing a channel through which the light of your essence can continue to flow in and the negativity you are working with can flow out.

7. EMBODY
Embody and externalize this healing by visualizing the light of your essence flowing into each cell of your body.

Part Four

On the
Road to
Healing

9

The 28-Day Healing Journey

INTRODUCTION TO THE JOURNEY

Unconditional love, joy, and inner peace are not simply goals to be pursued. They are our birthright, and we experience them when we let go of the conditioned thought patterns and illusion in our lives. We can *never* experience joy, unconditional love, and inner peace simply by pursuing them.

We need to remember that we are not our thoughts, and that our essence exists on some level without thought. Discovering our essence is not a pursuit. We cannot seek to discover or experience the truth that lies within our essence through effort or hard work. We may experience it, but we cannot seek it out. We can only begin to discover it by letting go of our ego—even for a few minutes. By ego, I mean the person we think we are—the ambitious, the successful, the honest, the brilliant. Our ego is always searching and seeking. It may find success, money, or possessions, but it will never find the truth that lies within our essence. The truth exists in the moment. It is there for us to discover: not tomorrow, but now.

Your essence exists. Its truth, insight, and perspective await your discovery. What must you let go of to discover this? The answer is obvious: If your mind is constantly focused on fears of the future, ambition, or worry about something in the past that cannot be changed, then it cannot also know the truth, insight, and perspective inherent in who you really are.

I want you to see how easy it is to let go of just one thing that you cling to. You can surrender this thing you cling to by *effortlessly* brushing it aside.

Have you ever for just one day let go of, say, your fear of the future? Just given it up without fear of what will happen to you, brushed it aside without anxiety, and without any struggle involving will power? Try it.

You can do this by letting go of one thing at a time. The ESSENCE meditation healing will reveal to you each day what you need to surrender or give up in your life in order to learn the truth of who you are. Just let go of one thing for one day; for example, ambition, or smoking, or worrying about the future. Say to yourself, "Just today, I simply brush aside my fear of the future. Today is enough for me. Whatever I am or am given today will be enough. Today, I allow this petty, conditioned thought pattern called my fear of the future to just die."

It can be put very simply in the following way. When I *am*, my ego is *not*. When my ego *is*, I am *not*.

If you can simply let go of whatever it is you choose, effortlessly and without force, you will discover what it means to live in the present moment. You will have lived a day from your essence and learned a great truth about yourself and your life.

All you need is a quiet mind and an open heart.

Healing is a journey, and when traveling it the ESSENCE way, you follow the four paths described in the preceding chapters. On the 28-Day Healing Journey, you spend a day at each step. Do only one step each day. Keep each step with you throughout the day, and refer to it as often as you feel necessary.

PATH I: HEALING FEAR

(Days 1–7)

The first ESSENCE healing path allows you to begin to see the fear in your life, and how different your life can be when you begin to release this fear. Each of the seven steps involved is designed to help you to focus on how ubiquitous fear has become in your life, and to guide you to see your own power to release that fear.

Day 1

STEP 1. EXPERIENCE

I will experience all fear today from the viewpoint of my essence, rather than just think about it with my mind.

Each time I think of a fear with my mind, I will stop and ask, "Can this fear hurt the reality of who I am? Is this fear outside of me, or am I creating it within my own thoughts?"

Visualize your entire physical life—from birth to death—as having a span of a single day. Now say to yourself, "My entire life is as one day and I will live as if today were my entire life." If you keep this in mind for only one day and live it as if it were true, you will begin to gain great insight and inner strength. You will begin to see that life is about truly experiencing the process rather than only trying to achieve a result.

Day 2

STEP 2. SEE

I will see all fear today from the viewpoint of my essence.

My fear thinks, "This occurrence will make my life fall apart."

But my essence asks, "Was my life ever meant to be the same each day? Wouldn't life be stale if it were the same, day in and day out?"

My fear asks, "Wouldn't it be awful if this adversity were to happen someday?"

But my essence answers, "I need not dwell on this catastrophe or that adversity. Doing that robs today of its richness, and my mind could easily think of a thousand more adversities if I knew the one I'm now dwelling on would never happen."

Day 3

STEP 3. SURRENDER

I will surrender to my essence my thoughts about what I fear.

My fear thinks, "I cannot face this adversity, for it can overcome me."

But my essence answers, "I surrender to the reality that change is always going to be integral to my life, as it is to all life. I can also surrender to the fact that if I can face and look directly at my fear from the viewpoint of my essence, the fear will disappear—like all illusions."

Day 4

STEP 4. EMPOWER

I will empower my life by remembering my essence.

I will remember that within my essence lies my power.

I will remember that what I fear cannot take from me that which I can never lose.

I will remember that I now can let go of the fear of never finding that which my essence has always possessed.

Day 5

STEP 5. NUTURE

Each time I become conscious of thoughts or actions based on fear, I will nurture the perspective and insight I am creating by remembering to ask myself, "Am I avoiding an issue in my life out of fear?" When I do, I only rob myself of experiences.

Day 6

STEP 6. CREATE

I will create today the following insight: To live fully, I need to allow my fear to die. I realize the pain associated with all my fears lies in my avoidance of them.

I will create perspective by seeing today that my fears are based on thought, rooted in either the past or the future. My essence has a reality that is not the product of thought.

I will remember, "When I am aware of my essence, fear cannot be a reality, and only peace can prevail in my life."

Day 7

STEP 7. EMBODY

I will embody the perspective and insight within my essence today.

I will realize, whenever I feel my fear, that fear no longer has power over me because I no longer have the need to avoid it.

Whenever fear comes up today, I will ask, "If I created my fear with thoughts, can fear disappear by changing my thoughts? If I am living from my essence, can fear still exist?"

PATH II: GOING BEYOND SUFFERING

(Days 8–14)

The second ESSENCE healing path allows you to examine those areas that cause suffering in your life, and begin to heal them. Each of the seven steps in this path helps you see the causes of suffering in your life, and gives you the perspective to begin healing them.

Day 8

STEP 1. EXPERIENCE

I will experience today that my choice for security in illusions is a choice to have suffering. Whenever I become upset, angry, or frustrated, I will examine what it is I am seeking that I cannot find.

Am I clinging to security, or am I now willing to *experience* life by allowing it to happen?

When I seek security in illusion rather than just let life happen, I suffer.

When I focus on my desires and ambitions and thus neglect the needs of my essence and my body, I suffer.

Day 9

STEP 2. SEE

I will see all areas of suffering today from the viewpoint of my essence.

Whenever I have pain associated with an unwanted reality today, I will ask, "Why do I find this unwanted reality so painful or frightening?"

I will also examine each painful aspect by asking, "To what degree do my thoughts about suffering cause me more suffering?"

I will then see these from the viewpoint of my essence, and realize that suffering has no power over me when I am aware of my essence.

Day 10

STEP 3. SURRENDER

I surrender to the healing that lies within my essence.

Today, I will surrender the painful thoughts associated with the causes of my suffering. I will examine honestly any lessons that may be here for me.

Today, I will just observe my life and realize that unwanted occurrences are a necessary part of my existence and are not inherently bad.

Day 11

STEP 4. EMPOWER

I will empower my life today by experiencing my essence.

My essence is who I really am. I am not my fear. I am not suffering. I am not my worries. I am not my ambition. I am not my success. I simply am. I have simple needs that I have been neglecting.

Today, I will listen to the needs of my essence and give them precedence over all the desires and worries of my ego.

Day 12

STEP 5. NURTURE

I will nurture the insight of my true reality by listening to the needs of my essence.

How have I been neglecting my essence? What haven't I been doing because I was afraid I would fail? What haven't I been doing because I was too busy trying to make a living or worrying about the future?

I will take time today to nurture my essence by first listening to it and then taking care of its needs.

Day 13

STEP 6. CREATE

I will create a new life by beginning to live based on the truth of who I am.

I have thought that I was my worries, ambition, and fear. My essence has the insight and perspective to bring a new simplicity based on truth to my life.

Today, I will give myself time to see the truths that lie within my essence, and I will begin to live them.

Day 14

STEP 7. EMBODY

I will embody the reality of my essence and the truths within me by living with an awareness of who I am.

When I see suffering, pain, and fear crop up today, I will ask, "Am I trying to be who I am not?"

I will take the time to see that my essence can understand all events in a way that frees me from suffering.

I will also take the time to see how much of my suffering I cause myself by ignoring the truths and needs within my essence.

PATH III: ENDING MELANCHOLY

(Days 15–21)

The third ESSENCE healing path allows you to begin to heal those areas of your life that cause sadness, melancholy, or depression. Each of the seven steps in this path helps you see the causes of sadness or depression in your life, and helps you gain the insight to begin healing them.

Day 15

STEP 1. EXPERIENCE

I will today experience those areas of sadness or sorrow in my life.

When I feel sadness, I will accept it and feel it fully.

Then I will ask, "Do these feelings originate within me or outside of me?"

Day 16

STEP 2. SEE

Today, I will see that areas where there is sadness begin within my own thoughts.

When I see my sadness from the viewpoint of my essence, I can let it be.

The more I can become one with my sadness and stop avoiding it, the less painful it will be.

I can thus use it to learn lessons, which is one of the major reasons I'm here in the first place.

What lessons can my sadness teach me when I accept it?

Day 17

STEP 3. SURRENDER

I will surrender my sadness, depression, and sorrow to my essence.

I will see that the feeling of acceptance and the lightness of letting go of my sadness are one and the same.

I will see today how I may use my sadness and my sorrow to learn lessons about life, as well as the truth of who I really am.

Day 18

STEP 4. EMPOWER

I will empower my life by healing my sadness and sorrow.

Today, I will remind myself, "I have the power and safety within my essence to experience and heal, rather than continue to avoid my sorrow."

Now that I know what avoidance of my sadness and sorrow feels like, I will imagine what acceptance and healing of it feel like.

Day 19

STEP 5. NURTURE

Today, I will nurture my acceptance of my sadness, as well as the perspective I have attained from seeing it from my essence.

I will remember throughout the day, "My sadness and sorrow were born out of forgetting, and now is the time to remember."

Day 20

STEP 6. CREATE

I will create my life now from my essence, which can only be free from sadness and sorrow.

My mind may always have some sadness, but I am not just my mind. My mind is here for me to use. I may use its sadness, but I will not become identified with it, because I will not forget who I am.

Day 21

STEP 7. EMBODY

Today, I will embody the vision of my life from the viewpoint of my essence.

I choose to have what I know I deserve: peace and harmony that come from the freedom of being totally identified with my mind's sadness.

I will feel deeply my desire to let go of the causes of sorrow in my life.

PATH IV: CREATING HOPE

(Days 22–28)

The fourth ESSENCE healing path allows you to see how destructive, negative explanations about your life originate in your mind and contribute to your suffering. Each of the seven steps in this path leads you toward the realization that healing and transformation are available to you when you move into your essence.

Day 22

STEP 1. EXPERIENCE

I will experience how I explain to myself today my illness (or another unwanted occurrence).

When I am thinking about an unwanted occurrence, I will stop and ask myself, "How am I explaining the meaning of this and its outcome?"

I will remind myself, "My explanations about this occurrence originate within me, even though I see this occurrence as having originated outside myself."

I will remind myself throughout the day, "I wish to experience what this occurrence means."

Day 23

STEP 2. SEE

Today, I will see how I am free to choose different, more constructive explanations aligned with my essence.

I will remind myself, "I am free to choose what I believe about this unwanted reality and my life. I can explain this and draw conclusions about it in a way that can bring hope and healing, rather than despair and fear."

I will further remind myself, "My outlook and explanations, which seem to be concrete and permanent, are actually nothing more than thoughts that can simply be released."

Day 24

STEP 3. SURRENDER

Today, I will surrender my negative outlook and explanations to my essence.

I will allow myself to see that there is a part of me that can be served by what I have been explaining only negatively.

I will remind myself, "I may be powerless to change the past, but I am no longer powerless to change my attitudes, thoughts, and outlook. I am no longer powerless to bring healing from my essence."

Day 25

STEP 4. EMPOWER

I empower myself to remove the barriers to healing. These barriers lie mostly in my thoughts and ego, and they block me from knowing the vast power that lies within my essence.

I will remind myself, "My outlook, attitude, and explanations are my reality now, but they are not based on truth. I realize this is a temporary reality, and I wish to create a new reality based within my essence. I trust in my power to transform conclusions, outlooks, and attitudes that do not serve me well."

Day 26

STEP 5. NURTURE

I will nurture and cultivate my new explanations by reminding myself throughout the day, "While I may not be able to control all events and circumstances in my life, I can control my attitudes, explanations, and conclusions about them. I choose to think about my life with constructive thoughts, and to heal it with all the power that lies within my essence."

Day 27

STEP 6. CREATE

I will create today a space where acceptance and transformation can continue. I can spend time in this space anytime I need to, and it is here that I am totally safe.

Day 28

STEP 7. EMBODY

Today, I will embody and actualize my transformation. I will remind myself, "I will continue on the path of acceptance, transformation, and healing. I will do this by living my life with an awareness of who I am. I will endeavor to learn my purpose and any lessons that are here for me today."

I will also remind myself, "When my explanations move me toward health, harmony, and fullfillment, they are used as intended by my essence."

ESSENCE healing must be regularly practiced, since it is only by continually experiencing life from the viewpoint of your soul that you can begin to live without fear and illusion. Do not become discouraged if you find yourself immersed again in worry or fear after having experienced peace and joy inside your heart. Know that each time you touch the reality of your essence, a part of you is healed. You will find that the more your life is lived based on the reality of who you are, the easier it becomes to embrace and live life fully. Allow yourself the freedom to stumble and make mistakes on your journey.

You are not perfect, which simply means you need to be open to learning the lessons necessary for your growth.

10

The Multiple Paths to Inner Life

In introducing the ESSENCE Guided Imagery meditations in the opening chapters of this book, I emphasized that they made up for things lacking in modern medicine. For the sake of simplicity, I barely touched on the great spiritual traditions from which these meditations originate. I would like to mention some aspects of these traditions that I have found particularly enlightening, and also some more contemporary approaches to releasing our inner powers.

EASTERN BELIEFS

The historical and present-day conflicts of Christians, Jews, and Muslims have helped give Eastern religions a tranquil, spiritual aura. Yoga and the various forms of Buddhism are attractive to many Westerners because they teach that other people do not have to be wrong for you to be right. In the way they are understood by Westerners, at least, yoga and Buddhism also seem to be more universal than our Western faiths. To most of us, our spiritual potential as individuals is more interesting than arguments about which particular group is specially favored by the Creator.

Yoga and Buddhism, however, remain stubbornly foreign and

exotic to Western culture, no matter how useful and sensible their concepts can be. Perhaps ways of expressing their central ideas will have to be changed almost out of recognition before they are popularly accepted. But, from a healer's point of view, being realistic about such cultural differences is important. An American physician familiar with the Ayurvedic medicine of India, for example, may see how it could help a particular patient. If this patient has lived all his life in Scranton, Pennsylvania, and his only knowledge of India is curry powder, he may have a strong resistance to the doctor's recommendation, regardless of its benefits. Similarly, suggesting a Buddhist practice to a devout Baptist woman in the South could actually increase her stress level and potentially damage her health. We Americans expect all-American health care, and yoga and Eastern meditation are not yet widely accepted as part of that care.

ACUPUNCTURE

Acupuncture strikes many twentieth-century people the same way yoga did nineteenth-century British soldiers—as strange and unworkable. Yet for many people acupuncture obviously does work. Typically used to relieve pain, it has also been successful in the treatment of anxiety, depression, drug and alcohol addiction, and other disorders.

In his book *Encounters with Qi*, the American physician David Eisenberg described how he witnessed brain surgery in Beijing performed with acupuncture as the anesthetic. The fifty-eight-year-old patient had a chestnut-sized tumor at the pituitary gland. The surgeon had to approach it by cutting a hole through the top of the skull. The patient—a college professor who had his own doubts about acupuncture!—was given a mild preoperative sedative by the anesthesiologist. She then inserted needles beneath the skin at six acupuncture points of his body: on each eyebrow, at two points on his right temple, and on his left shin and ankle. At intervals, she stimulated the needles with a low-voltage battery. As she manipulated the needles, she asked the patient, "Do you have qi?" She meant by this whether he had a feeling of fullness, distention, and mild electric shock at the points being stimulated. "I have it," he assured her.

The patient was awake throughout the surgical procedure, which took more than four hours. He felt pressure, but no pain. When the operation was finished, he sat up on the table, shook hands with the neurosurgeon and anesthesiologist, and thanked them. If he had been in New York instead of Beijing, he would have been an instant television sensation. Proponents of acupuncture believe it works through the needles balancing or freeing the flow of *qi* (pronounced *chee* and also frequently spelled *chi*). Qi is believed to circulate through the body along twelve meridians or pathways, each of which is linked to a particular organ or organ system. Researchers have tried to find physical evidence of meridians in the body, so far without any widely accepted success. Some have considered qi a liquid and have searched for ducts that might conduct it. Others have regarded it as an electricity-like form of energy. I think it's reasonable to speculate that it might be the ancient Chinese equivalent of what other cultures see as an inner healing power, or spiritual force, or even the Judeo-Christian soul.

Chinese culture is unique in two ways: it's far older than any other currently existing culture and, until the twentieth century, it seems to have changed less over enormous lengths of time than any other culture. Poems written more than three thousand years ago are in the same tradition as those written only a hundred years ago. Acupuncture is thought to be more than five thousand years old. Perhaps some of our mystification is due to an ancient way of presenting knowledge, as well as to cultural differences.

For example, if Hippocrates were to address an American Medical Association conference in, say, New Orleans later this year, he would probably impress most of the doctors there with the accuracy of his clinical observation of symptoms. However, his explanation of these symptoms would suddenly place him at a distance of many centuries. And the explanations of qi go back even further in time than the ancient Greeks.

I refer again to Dr. Eisenberg's account for how the modern Chinese visualize qi. The possession of qi distinguishes animate things from the inanimate, and the living from the dead. A dead body has no qi. Good health depends on a balance of qi. Either too much or too little qi causes ill health. This sense of balance of qi is strikingly similar to the homeostasis concept of Cannon (chapter 5) in that both schools of thought seek equilibrium of the mind/body. So too, in their own terminology, do the masters of yoga.

How does a doctor put all that into conversational English? I say, "Try to lead a *harmonious* life." Without any of the preceding discussion, many people know exactly what I mean.

BIOENERGETICS AND VISUALIZATION

Several years ago, I began using bioenergetics with cancer patients. We used biofeedback, meditation, and visualization to deal with their fears, worries, and pain. I felt it would be useful to find a way to merge the benefits of focusing, core energetics, and visualization/meditation. Focusing helps you notice where in your body your emotions are localized. Core energetics is a way of finding emotional blocks localized in the body. Visualization and meditation help you achieve the relaxation response, help free you from feelings of helplessness, and help give you a positive attitude that can benefit the immune system.

One August afternoon at a swimming pool, I noticed I had a very faint, tiny, brownish mole on the sole of my right foot. Even though it was hardly visible, and I was not sure it had not always been there, I made an appointment to see a prominent dermatologist in New York. He carefully examined the mole and assured me it was nothing to worry about. I told him my concern that melanomas (skin cancers) occurring in this area are among the most aggressive and fatal. He assured me it was not a melanoma and suggested I observe it and see him again in three or four months. I felt relieved.

Eight weeks later, at a workshop on bioenergetics, I was meditating and became aware of a coldness and tingling in my right foot. I warmed my foot, massaged it, and exercised to relieve it. Over the next twenty-four hours, the sensation increased. During another meditation, I came to know with the deepest intuitive conviction that the mole was about to become malignant. To my naked eye, it looked no different than before.

The following day I made an appointment to see the dermatologist again. He examined the mole with a magnifying glass, and his words confirmed my inner knowing: "Oh my God, it's really changed—it's irregular, larger, and darker. I have to take it off immediately."

The lesion turned out to be a markedly atypical mole, but not yet melanoma. The dermatologist said that it was rapidly degenerating and that I was very lucky to have come back in early.

My primary interest in bioenergetics was to help cancer patients. I had never expected I would need to make use of it myself.

FOCUSING

Alternative psychological therapies make use of our inner healing power to varying extents. Focusing appeals directly to it. While its adherents are likely to use a different terminology than mine, focusing could be described as a way of establishing a conscious mind/body connection. It requires practice and a certain amount of know-how.

As described by the psychologist Eugene T. Gendlin in his book *Focusing*, six steps are involved:

1. Clearing a space—listen inwardly to your body.
2. Felt sense—select your biggest problem.
3. Finding a handle—think of a single word that best describes the quality of your problem, such as *helpless* or *burdened.*
4. Resonating handle and felt sense—think of the word and your problem together.
5. Asking—consider why the problem makes you feel, for example, helpless or burdened.
6. Receiving—welcome whatever insight you are given.

I reached the broad conclusion, from studying my patients, that there are many ways to put our inner healing power to use, in focusing, for example. Some ways are more effective than others. Some work better for one kind of personality than another. The sole criterion has to be: if it heals, use it.

Cigarettes, alcohol, and drugs may help relieve stress or lift depression to varying degrees, but for a very short time. None are nearly as powerful or long-lasting as putting your inner healing power to use.

GUIDED IMAGERY

American therapist Belleruth Naparstek defined *guided imagery* as a kind of directed daydreaming. Her book *Staying Well with Guided Imagery* provides a wealth of information on the subject for the general reader. The imagery is not restricted to visual images. Sights, sounds, smells, tastes, touch, and various physical sensations may be more evocative for some people.

Our mind has a beneficial influence on our body when it is free of stress and filled with tranquil thoughts. Our body does not question whether such thoughts are justifiable; it accepts them. Therefore, even though the "events" of guided imagery are not real events, they have real physical benefits.

Strengthening the immune system is among these real physical benefits. Claims that guided imagery can benefit the immune system have been supported by studies by Nicholas Hall at the George Washington University Medical Center, by Frank Lawlis at the University of Texas, by C. Wayne Smith and John Schneider at Michigan State University, and by Karen Olness at the Children's Hospital in Cleveland. Other studies have shown that guided imagery can replace histamine as a treatment for poison ivy and can reduce pain, stress, and depression.

People who enter a euphoric state through guided imagery seem to increase their powers of healing, learning, and change while in that state. Some people also achieve this state by using breathing techniques.

PRAYER

In modernizing the rituals of the Roman Catholic church, the Second Vatican Council (1962–1965) dropped the use of Gregorian chant. At about the time this decision was made, the French physician Alfred Tomatis visited a Benedictine monastery in France. He noticed the general good health of the monks there, who rose before dawn, lived on a vegetarian diet, and spent hours every day praying and chanting together in their church.

In February 1967, Dr. Tomatis was asked to return to the monastery because seventy of the ninety-seven monks there were listless and having health problems. On seeing that these complaints were true, the doctor turned detective. What was happening here now that was not happening on his previous visit, when everyone had been so healthy? The monks were getting more sleep, they were eating meat, and they no longer spent hours chanting every day.

The doctor's recommendation was simple. They were to go back to the way that monks had been living for seven hundred years before the change—less sleep, no meat, and lots of chanting. In less than nine months, the monks were their old selves again.

Gregorian chant is a form of prayer. Even psychiatrists who do not believe in a Supreme Being recognize that someone who believes can gain much release from stress through prayer. Chanting is something you do with other people; this creates a feeling of fellowship and common interest, which also reduces stress. In fact, with wrong notes, sneezes, and comical mistakes, monks with a sense of humor probably have a lot of fun chanting! In addition, monks pray not for their own personal needs but for the benefit of humankind. This magnanimity toward others adds purpose and joy—both great stress reducers—to their lives.

That's from a Western point of view. Someone with an Eastern point of view might remark that Gregorian chant is equivalent to chanting mantra. Chanting mantra helps create a mind-set that rejects what it regards as negative thoughts. This mind-set helps create a harmonious balance between the mind, emotions, and body. This, of course, is the kind of integration most readily identified with healing.

One of my own greatest assists toward prayer was not strictly religious at all, but was the book *The Road Less Traveled*, by the psychiatrist M. Scott Peck. This book, which I first read as a fourth-year medical student, is well on its way to becoming a classic, and it has recently been followed by Peck's *Further along the Road Less Traveled*.

SHAMANISM

Much nonsense has been written about shamanism, but there is much that is authentic about this ancient tradition. Shamans are holy people who are said to have magical powers of healing, divination, or control. Their methods are similar in societies all over the world: they are reported to use invisible spiritual powers to achieve visible physical results. Some invoke gods, ancestral spirits, or nature spirits; they may use fire, special objects, hallucinogens, alcohol, or medicinal plants. They may or may not have a powerful personal presence, but most inspire fear and respect.

A shaman's procedures would make most Americans somewhat cynical. But even if we are unlikely to find shamans widely accepted in the near future, we need not overlook their abilities as healers. A sick person who has been cured by a shaman is little bothered whether academic authorities regard his or her sickness and cure as acceptable.

One of the extraordinary things about shamanism is that it seems not to need the cooperation of the person to be healed. One crusty old gentleman, the father of a friend of mine, found that his arthritis was relieved when he wore a copper bracelet given him by a rural Irish woman who was famed as a healer. Nevertheless, he refused to acknowledge its healing power. Wearing the bracelet only when his condition became painful, he always hid it beneath a shirt sleeve. If someone noticed it, he laughed it off as superstitious nonsense his wife had foisted on him, and as something he wore only to please her. But although it went against everything he believed, it never once failed.

From time to time, patients show me a charm, amulet, or other device given to them as a good-health talisman. I encourage them to wear it, just so long as they *add* wearing the talisman to things they are already doing. Also, they should not use it to replace some healing procedure they do not like.

Michael Lerner, in *Choices in Healing*, stresses that a shaman's greatest concern is safeguarding the patient's soul. His or her function is to bring the soul back to life, if that is meant to be; if it is not, the shaman tries to conduct the soul safely to the next world. The patient's physical welfare is of secondary concern. This is actually not far from the viewpoint of some Americans' down-home, old-time religion. Most of us would hesitate before seeing a physician whom we knew to hold such views. But someone who is familiar with the frontier between life and death, and who is unafraid of it, can give strength and hope to an ailing person and can permit that person to make maximum use of his or her inner healing force. Another "old-fashioned virtue" of shamanism is that it, like all great spiritual traditions, accepts pain as an aid to enlightenment. Nowadays we argue vociferously against such platitudes and consume painkillers in extraordinary quantities.

Lerner describes how most modern medical doctors, equipped with every instrument for technical care, have never been on the edge of death themselves. They worry about a patient developing false hopes from what they say. For many physicians, trained for a can-do and fix-it world, communicating with a patient's deep inner powers sounds like something out of science fiction.

If shamanism is even more exotic—and out of the question—for most of us than yoga or Buddhism, it still presents us with a glaring need. We need to recognize that hope may be as important as an IV, that purpose may be as important as a hospital bed, and that fellowship means more than medical insurance.

YOGA

In the nineteenth century, British colonial administrators and soldiers in India reported home about the wonders performed by mystics and holymen. Many of them were masters of yoga, which is an ancient offshoot of Hinduism. Their seemingly impossible physical feats and resistance to pain could make hardened military men wince. Experts back in Britain dismissed these displays as tricks played by wily natives on good-hearted but simple-minded soldiers. But the stories persisted, and in time were backed by photographs.

Some of these demonstrations may indeed have been tricks. But yoga masters have repeatedly shown a mind-over-body control that has amazed Western anatomists and physiologists, creating in the Western mind a greater fascination for yoga than for other Hindu and Muslim spiritual disciplines. These feats are physical and visible; we are much less intrigued by emotional and invisible wonders.

For its practitioners, yoga is no series of circus tricks. *Yoga* means "union," referring to the integration of mental, emotional, and spiritual powers. When the mind and emotions are in a disturbed state, it is believed that physical health is at risk. Conversely, when a person is physically sick, thought is believed to be less clear. Yoga exercises and meditations evolved to take care of both physical and emotional disorders. They were first described in writing more than two thousand years ago.

An incident from the 1890s illustrates the power a calm mind is believed to have over the body. The follower of a famous Bengali guru was badly bitten by a deadly asp. The man had only hours to live, during which time the guru meditated with him. Skilled in meditation, the stricken man followed the guru's spiritual directions, and within days, he completely recovered. Two years later, however, this man was agitating politically against the British presence in India. He became involved in an argument, lost his temper, and dropped dead. His autopsy revealed he had died from asp venom. Of course, it's possible that he was bitten by a second asp. But yoga adepts believe that the meditation of a tranquil mind, at a very high level of discipline, is a match even for deadly snake venom.

Various aspects of yoga make it very accessible to Westerners. You need only go as far as you wish; there is no compulsion to move on to another level. It does not run counter to most religious beliefs and civil duties, and there is no demand to join a cult or shave your head. But you do have to overcome some strange terms and concepts at the beginning, which unfortunately scares people off. As a physician, I have to tread carefully in recommending yoga to people who have been conditioned to expect help from a medicine bottle.

11

Nutrients and Cancer

Cancer is now the leading cause of death for American women. If current trends continue, it will become the leading cause of death for both men and women by the year 2000. This does not mean that the incidence of cancer is rising at an explosive rate. In fact, from 1950 to 1987, it increased by only 6 percent. Here were the estimated leading causes of American deaths in 1990:

Heart and blood vessel diseases	930,500
Cancer	506,000
Accidents	93,600
Chronic obstructive pulmonary disease	78,600
All other causes	464,300

Source: National Center for Health Statistics and American Heart Association.

Cancer's rise to prominence as the leading cause of death in the United States will depend on a continuing decline in the incidence of cardiovascular disease, the current leading cause. Less fatty diets and more exercise have helped reduce the nation's coronary death rate by 40 percent since 1968. If increasing numbers of Americans adopt healthy lifestyles in the next few years, cardiovascular disease will be affected accordingly.

The challenge, therefore, is not how to control cancer as some raging ogre out of control in a ravaged environment, which undeniably makes for a graphic presentation. The real question is whether we Americans can do to cancer what we have succeeded in doing to cardiovascular disease.

I believe Americans can dramatically reduce their incidence of cancer. Part of that effort will rely on the synthesis of new wonder drugs and on high-tech surgery, as has been true in the fight against heart disease. And, as with heart disease, a major part of the prevention program will consist of people taking control of their own health destiny. One of the major ways to do that is through diet.

Diet can be directly associated with colon/rectal and stomach cancers, which made up 15 percent and 2 percent, respectively, of new American cancer cases in 1990. A diet high in animal fat and low in fiber contributes to colon/rectal cancer. The role of fat and fiber in the development of cancer has been studied extensively.

The prevention of approximately another fifth of cancers is within our control. These are cancers caused by environmental factors, such as ultraviolet light from the sun, trauma of many kinds, X-rays, and drugs. We have to face facts: tobacco and dietary animal fat cause about half of all cancer cases in America today. We can certainly do something about that!

One of the most important things we can do is to make sure our food contains certain nutrients that taste pleasant, are easy to find, and don't cost much. By taking reasonable precautions against cancer, cardiovascular disease, and accidents, we can prolong our lives beyond anything thought possible only a few decades ago. Not only do we gain in *quantity* of life, but our continuing good health ensures that we gain in *quality* of life also.

PEOPLE WITH A HIGHER RISK OF CANCER

When looking at the incidence of cancer, we are really dealing with two groups of people: first, the general population and, second, people who have a higher risk of developing cancer than the general population. The latter group is at higher risk of cancer for four reasons:

1. Engaging in personal behaviors such as smoking and heavy drinking
2. Being genetically predisposed to malignancy
3. Already having an illness that often results in cancer
4. Having biomarkers (lab tests) indicative of a higher risk of developing cancer

Unregulated cell division, which characterizes cancer, possibly has many causes. In all likelihood, three of the most frequent causes are DNA damage, cell membrane damage, and an impaired immune system.

DNA DAMAGE

We return again to high school biology class to recall that our genes lie along a double helix of DNA within the nucleus of each cell. Damage to the DNA (from a virus or X-rays, for example) may alter its "message" or help activate undesirable genes. A cell with damaged DNA may divide into new mutant cells. The body may not have the means to control further division of these strange new cells, and thus their growth will be unregulated.

CELL MEMBRANE DAMAGE

Substances can damage the cell membrane, which is the permeable and flexible outer wall of a human cell. Besides allowing chemical messages to seep into and out of the cell, the membrane itself contains sensors to detect them. Damage to membrane sensors may send haywire messages to the cell nucleus, and this may indirectly affect rapid cell division.

IMPAIRED IMMUNE SYSTEM

A healthy immune system recognizes and destroys damaged or mutant cells in the bloodstream. If the immune system is compromised in some way, it may not be able to do so. This could permit the abnormal cells to develop into cancer.

THE CANCER PROCESS

What might appear to be cell anarchy is actually a process that always involves a number of steps, all of which must be completed before fully developed cancer gets under way. The more steps a process involves, of course, the greater the number of opportunities to halt it.

The cancer process can be simplified into the following sequence of steps:

Precarcinogen/Carcinogen ⟶ Initiation ⟶
Promotion ⟶ Progression ⟶
Cancer ⟶ Metastasis

PRECARCINOGENS AND CARCINOGENS

Any agent that starts the cancer process is a carcinogen. Chemicals, certain viruses, and radiation are examples of environmental carcinogens. Precarcinogens are agents that need to be altered in some way, usually within the body, before they can act as carcinogens.

INITIATION

The initial injury to the body cell that gets the process under way is called initiation. DNA damage is an example.

PROMOTION

Agents that encourage the precancerous cells to divide are called promoters, and promotion is the stage during which such agents are most active. Alcohol, polyunsaturated fats, and some hormones are known to be effective promoters.

PROGRESSION

Progression can be thought of as the stage when the new, rapidly dividing cells establish themselves as a rebel colony within the body. They do this by setting up their own oxygen and glucose supply systems through the bloodstream. The main enemy of the new cells at this stage ought to be the immune system.

CANCER

The term *cancer* is used loosely. As a stage in the process, it usually indicates the formation of a tumor.

METASTASIS

The metastasis stage is when the cancer cells spread to other parts of the body.

BLOCKING AGENTS

Almost all carcinogens in food require metabolic activation. That is, the carcinogens remain inert unless they are triggered by a chemical or by special conditions. Blocking agents, also in our food, can prevent them from becoming active in a cancerous way.

The blocking agents occur in several kinds of vegetables. They are found in cruciferous vegetables, such as cabbage, broccoli, brussels sprouts, turnips, and mustard greens. Garlic is rich in sulfur-containing blocking agents, as are its relatives such as onions, leeks, and shallots. Citrus fruit oils contain another kind of blocking agent, two of which have been investigated. These are D-limonene and D-carvone. The latter is found also in caraway seed oil.

After being eaten in food, the above agents increase the activity of the detoxifying, or so-called phase II, enzymes. Enzymes help reactions take place without becoming involved themselves. Phase II enzymes facilitate reactions that break down active carcinogens in the body before they can damage the DNA of cells. These substances are broken down into harmless detoxification products, which are then used in other processes or eliminated from the body.

Phase I enzymes also detoxify cancer-causing compounds. The drawback of phase I enzymes is that as well as detoxifying some substances, they may cause some benign compounds to become carcinogens. This means that nutrients that decrease the activity of phase I enzymes should also be included in a cancer-prevention diet. Green teas and garlic may do this.

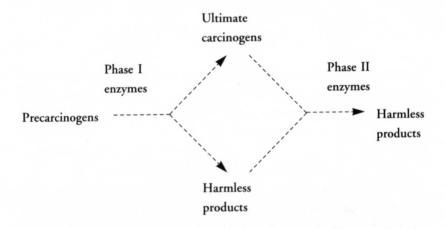

Many blocking agents protect cells by trapping oxygen-free radicals or preventing their formation. In this way, they act as antioxidants. Free radicals are unstable molecules that readily join with other molecules to form new substances, some of which may be injurious to cells. In the free radical theory of aging, these molecules are held responsible for much cell damage over time, causing organs to become vulnerable to disease. Antioxidants, such as vitamins C and E, link up with the free radicals to form harmless compounds.

SUPPRESSING AGENTS

Suppressing agents stop the development of damaged cells, and thus suppress the growth of what would have turned out to be cancerous tissue. How suppressing agents work can only be guessed at, and much less is known about them than about blocking agents.

Not many suppressing agents have been identified. Some occur in cruciferous vegetables. When we know more about them, we may find they are much more plentiful and widespread than we now know.

At Strang, we are studying common carcinogens in the environment. Of most interest to us are those found in our food.

ANTICANCER NUTRIENTS

According to a March 1994 paper in the *Journal of the National Cancer Institute*, of people living in a region of China with a high rate of esophageal cancer, those who drank green tea daily had only half as much esophageal cancer as those who did not. A 1991 *American Journal of Epidemiology* paper showed that low levels of vitamins A, C, and E were associated with an increased risk for developing stomach, colon/rectal, and lung cancers.

Three-quarters of the world population relies on plants and plant extracts for medicine. More than a hundred prescription drugs are derived from plants, and almost three-quarters of them came to the attention of pharmaceutical companies because of their use in folk medicine. The chemotherapy "wonder drugs" taxol, velban, and vincristine are examples. At Strang, we scientifically examine herbs, algae, mushrooms, antioxidants, teas, and garlic for their properties in cancer prevention and treatment.

As noted in the *Journal of Urology*, in a study of men with early-stage bladder cancer, all were treated with BCG instilled into the bladder (a method of boosting the immune system to fight the disease). One group was treated with BCG alone, and a second group also received high doses of vitamins A, B_6, C, and E. About 80 percent of the men treated with BCG alone had recurrent cancer, in contrast to about 40 percent of the men treated with BCG plus vitamins.

As noted before, a diet rich in cruciferous vegetables results in a decreased incidence of cancer. Dr. Leon Bradlow, at Strang, has done pioneering research on indol-3-carbinol, a substance found in cruciferous vegetables that increases the body's production of a protective estrogen called 2-hydroxy estrone. Indol-3-carbinol has already been shown to protect lab animals against breast cancer, and studies with humans are in progress.

With other Strang researchers, I am engaged in a study of alterations in biomarkers of carcinogenesis associated with a high intake of cruciferous vegetables. Cruciferous vegetables also contain another recently identified compound, sulforaphane, which blocks the growth of tumors in rats exposed to carcinogens. This compound is able to increase certain detoxifying or phase II enzymes as well. Sulforaphane is just one of a whole class of chemicals, found in vegetables, called isothiocyanates. These so-called phytochemicals are able to enhance the body's own ability to ward off cancer.

Examples of other phytochemicals are allyl sulfides, which are found in garlic, onions, leeks, and chives. These compounds may block the action of certain carcinogens. Soybeans and other dried beans contain isoflavones (which may block estrogen from entering cells, potentially decreasing the risk of breast and ovarian cancer), phytosterols (which hinder cell division in the gut, possibly preventing colon cancer), and saponins (which prevent cancer cells from multiplying). Citrus fruits contain limonene, which increases detoxifying enzymes, while other fruits contain caffeic acid (which also increases detoxifying enzymes) and ferulic acid, which binds to nitrites, possibly preventing carcinogenesis. The science of nutrition's role in cancer prevention and treatment will continue to provide wonderful tools for all of us to use in the fight against cancer.

A Final Word

Imagination serves as the homeopathic elixir that heals; the practice of such healing requires that one experience the soul of the outer world through one's inner eye of soul.
—*Robert Sardello*,
FACING THE WORLD WITH SOUL

This book was not written as a "how-to" manual or as a way to convince you that any particular philosophy or religion is right or wrong. My intent is to allow you to see how the unconscious plays a prominent role not just in illness but in every aspect of our lives. I also wish for you to begin to sense your essential power and to develop an awareness of your essence, to ask yourself whether you may be here for more than just to work and struggle, and to begin to listen to the longings and yearnings that come forth. Devote time to this process, and act on the feelings and realizations that come to you. As noted earlier at various points, many people find it helpful to keep a journal to record this process.

Our unconscious has many aspects. Some aspects may choose death or illness to resolve conflicts or learn certain lessons. I described Mary, who developed cancer after the loss of her daughter when the "mother" part of her unconscious could not imagine life without her. We saw how Dave's focus on the "power" aspect of his unconscious reacted when faced with an illness that made him confront the lifetime of isolation his "power" had created. I have seen how a change in consciousness can alter the course of an illness. I have seen how acceptance can bring solace where there was dread. I have seen how surrender can empower people to find real healing.

You have long been searching, on some level, for the key to open the door behind which lies your inner power and healing. ESSENCE Guided Imagery allows this search to end. By surrendering, you learn how to open your life to the beauty and power of your essence. The sixth-century B.C. Chinese philosopher Lao Tzu once wrote:

> The universe is deathless,
> Is deathless because, having no finite self,
> It stays infinite.
> A sound man by not advancing himself
> Stays the further ahead of himself,
> By not confining himself to himself
> Sustains himself outside himself:
> By never being an end in himself
> He endlessly becomes himself.

You can surrender only when you know your essence, and only then can you have true healing. Until you attain this awareness, you will continue to react unconsciously to events rather than to exercise true choice. You will react out of fear rather than out of love, and continue to resist rather than surrender. Until you rediscover your essence, life will continue to teach you this lesson, until you finally learn it. These lessons may seem like senseless, painful events, until you learn their purpose.

Healing can result in the restoration of health, or it can bring about a realization of a lost part of you. It can bring about the surrender of illusions and fear, as well as the discovery of your essence. Healing of illness can lead to considerable possibilities. True healing, however, must occur in a context of forgiveness, which allows you to accept the imperfections of your body and those in your life.

As you begin to heal your fears and they begin to drop away, you see the power and light that you have been unaware of for so long. The initial joy people experience with this discovery often leads temporarily to an awareness of a deeper pain and suffering. I've noticed often with my patients that this pain is usually a mourning for the years of life they suddenly realize have slipped by, due to their fear and unawareness of who they really are.

You may also mourn the sudden shattering and loss of many of your old values. You will see that so many things you thought were important and real have simply been illusions with no lasting value or meaning to your essence. The hours one man spent working to advance his career are now seen as far less important than the years of missing his children's school plays and baseball games. The good times you wasted worrying about the future are now seen in the context of your essence—and you wonder how you could have never before known the effortlessness of living in harmony with who you really are. You ask how you could have ever done anything other than simply be open to life.

Be conscious of this mourning process. You can heal it by remembering that many people live their entire lives never knowing a moment of the true joy that comes from experiencing their essence. This transformation often takes many years, so that there is no need to dwell on the life that you have already allowed to slip by, the people you have hurt, and the opportunities you have lost. These were all lessons and necessary mistakes to bring you the awareness of how you have been living out of alignment with the truth of who you are. Surrender can continue to heal as you realize that while you cannot change the past, you can let go of its grip over your thoughts and your life. You may then begin to celebrate the healing, power, and joy that are now available to you.

Healing requires the openness to realize there may well be conflicts to be resolved or lessons to be learned from anything that causes discord in your life. Healing also requires a willingness to make the necessary transformation, so that this change can occur in place of an illness, depression, or other cause of pain. This is a truth most of us do not consider possible. We still put this in the realm of miracles. I have witnessed this so many times that I assure you it is not a miracle. Rather, healing is a gift of life that has been made available to all of us. But it is available only by becoming conscious of that which is now unconscious and by coming to know the truth of our essence and its power.

When we begin to understand our bodies and the world from beyond our mechanical point of view, the endless possibilities of healing come to light. Healing is truly never distant from the nature of the world or ourselves, and ESSENCE Guided Imagery can help us find and nurture that awareness.

Background Reading

American Psychiatric Association. *Diagnostic and Statistical Manual of Mental Disorders.* 4th ed. Washington, D.C.: American Psychiatric Association, 1994.

Borysenko, Joan. *Minding the Body, Mending the Mind.* Reading, Mass.: Addison-Wesley, 1987.

Buber, Martin. *Tales of the Hasidim.* New York: Schocken Books, 1991.

———. *Ten Rungs: Hasidic Sayings.* New York: Schocken Books, 1962.

Burton Goldberg Group. *Alternative Medicine: The Definitive Guide.* Puyallup, Wash.: Future Medicine, 1993.

Bynner, Witter. *The Chinese Translations.* New York: Farrar, Straus & Giroux, 1978.

Chuang Tzu. See Merton, Thomas.

Crick, Francis. *The Astonishing Hypothesis: The Scientific Search for the Soul.* New York: Scribner's, 1994.

Dickinson, Emily. *Complete Poems.* Boston: Little, Brown, 1960.

Eisenberg, David. *Encounters with Qi: Exploring Chinese Medicine.* New York: Norton, 1985.

Gendlin, Eugene T. *Focusing.* Rev. ed. New York: Bantam, 1981.

Goddard, Dwight, ed. *A Buddhist Bible.* Boston: Beacon, 1994.

Goodman, Berney. *When the Body Speaks Its Mind: A Psychiatrist Probes the Mysteries of Hypochondria, Somatization, and Munchausen's Syndrome.* New York: Tarcher/ Putnam, 1994.

Jung, C. G. *Modern Man in Search of a Soul.* New York: Harcourt, Brace & World, 1933.

Kabat-Zinn, Jon. *Wherever You Go, There You Are: Mindfulness Meditation in Everyday Life.* New York: Hyperion, 1994.

Keller, Helen. *The Story of My Life.* Garden City, N.Y.: Doubleday, 1954.

Laing, R. D. *The Divided Self.* New York: Pantheon, 1969.

Lao Tzu. See *The Chinese Translations* by Witter Bynner.

Lazarus, Richard S., and Susan Folkman. *Stress, Appraisal, and Coping.* New York: Springer, 1984.

Lerner, Max. *Wrestling with the Angel.* New York: Touchstone, 1990.

Lerner, Michael. *Choices in Healing: Integrating the Best of Conventional and Complementary Approaches to Cancer.* Cambridge, Mass.: MIT Press, 1994.

LeShan, Lawrence. *Cancer as a Turning Point: A Handbook for People with Cancer, Their Families, and Health Professionals.* Rev. ed. New York: Plume, 1994.

Locke, Steven, and Douglas Colligan. *The Healer Within: The New Medicine of Mind and Body.* New York: Dutton, 1986.

Maslow, Abraham H. *Toward a Psychology of Being.* 2d ed. Princeton, N.J.: Van Nostrand, 1968.

Merton, Thomas. *The Way of Chuang Tzu.* Boston: Shambhala, 1992.

Naparstek, Belleruth. *Staying Well with Guided Imagery.* New York: Warner, 1994.

Peck, M. Scott. *The Road Less Traveled.* New York: Simon & Schuster, 1979.

———. *Further along the Road Less Traveled.* New York: Simon & Schuster, 1993.

Pierrakos, John C. *Core Energetics: Developing the Capacity to Love and Heal.* Mendocino, Calif.: Life Rhythm, 1987.

Plotkin, Mark J. *Tales of a Shaman's Apprentice: An Ethnobotanist Searches for New Medicines in the Amazon Rain Forest.* New York: Penguin, 1993.

Reich, Wilhelm. *The Invasion of Compulsory Sex-Morality.* New York: Farrar, Straus & Giroux, 1971.

Rinpoche, Sogyal. *The Tibetan Book of Living and Dying.* San Francisco: HarperSanFrancisco, 1993.

Siegel, Bernie S. *Love, Medicine and Miracles.* New York: Harper & Row, 1986.

Simonton, O. Carl, and Reid Henson. *The Healing Journey.* New York: Bantam, 1992.

Suzuki, D. T. *Introduction to Zen.* New York: Grove/Atlantic, 1987.

For further information about ESSENCE Guided Imagery classes and audiovisual materials, please write to:

E.G.I., Inc.
Planetarium Station
P.O. Box 33
New York, NY
10024